The Art of Reiki
Developing Your Abilities
for Energy Healing

ARIANA WEBER

Copyright © 2019 Ariana Weber

All rights reserved.

ISBN: 9781701825932

This Book is provided with the sole purpose of providing relevant information on a specific topic for which every reasonable effort has been made to ensure that it is both accurate and reasonable. Nevertheless, by purchasing this Book you consent to the fact that the author, as well as the publisher, are in no way experts on the topics contained herein, regardless of any claims as such that may be made within. As such, any suggestions or recommendations that are made within are done so purely for entertainment value. It is recommended that you always consult a professional prior to undertaking any of the advice or techniques discussed within. This is a legally binding declaration that is considered both valid and fair by both the Committee of Publishers Association and the American Bar Association and should be considered as legally binding within the United States. The reproduction, transmission, and duplication of any of the content found herein, including any specific or extended information will be done as an illegal act regardless of the end form the information ultimately takes. This includes copied versions of the work both physical, digital and audio unless express consent of the Publisher is provided beforehand. Any additional rights reserved. Furthermore, the information that can be found within the pages described forthwith shall be considered both accurate and truthful when it comes to the recounting of facts. As such, any use, correct or incorrect, of the provided information will render the Publisher free of responsibility as to the actions taken outside of their direct purview. Regardless, there are zero scenarios where the original author or the Publisher can be deemed liable in any fashion for any damages or hardships that may result from any of the information discussed herein. Additionally, the information in the following pages is intended only for informational purposes and should thus be thought of as universal. As befitting its nature, it is presented without assurance regarding its prolonged validity or interim quality. Trademarks that are mentioned are done without written consent and can in no way be considered an endorsement from the trademark holder.

CONTENTS

	Introduction	1
1	Reiki History and Importance	5
2	Reiki Fundamentals	15
3	Understanding Your Psychic Gifts	37
4	Safe Psychic Development	61
5	Spiritual Perfection and Reiki	75
6	The Future of Reiki	105
7	Reiki Practice - Session Preparation	115
8	The Reiki Healing Session	127
9	Strengthen your Reiki with Crystals	149
10	Reiki – Bibliography	187
	Conclusion	191

INTRODUCTION

Our world, the reality surrounding us, is supported by a constantly fluctuating, flowing and endless life energy. She created the Cosmos, she also filled outer space. The existence of cosmic energy was known in antiquity. Ancient sages and scientists believed that there is the earthly energy of life and the original life energy. The first is formed from foods that the digestive system processes. A person receives the initial vital energy with his soul when he comes to this world. Strong life energy means that a person has powerful defenses - good immunity. The lack of vital energy results in weak immunity, susceptibility to various diseases, premature aging and death.

The goal of many spiritual practices (qigong, tai chi, yoga, etc.) is to slow down the trends of imbalance. Since disease in the interpretation of medicine is a blockage of the flow of vital energy, then by removing the blocks in the energy pathways that nourish the organs of the body (as well as muscles and ligaments), balance is restored. This allows the body to eliminate disharmony and improve health.

It is no coincidence that in modern China - a country with a millennium-old tradition of using special exercises that promote the circulation of vital energy - people of all ages perform exercises on open areas. And it is no coincidence that the regular execution of movements in combination with meditations allow a person to remain flexible in his body and mind in extreme old age. However, Chinese and Indian masters, as well as Reiki masters, not only developed a system of exercises but also cultivated the ability to arouse vital energy in other people.

It is worth emphasizing, though, the uniqueness of Reiki art, which consists in the fact that the transfer of the healing power of vital energy is possible only through the Reiki channel. If it is open, then transferring healing energy to others, as well as healing oneself, becomes easy and simple.

You are about to learn all about this!

REIKI

1 REIKI HISTORY AND IMPORTANCE

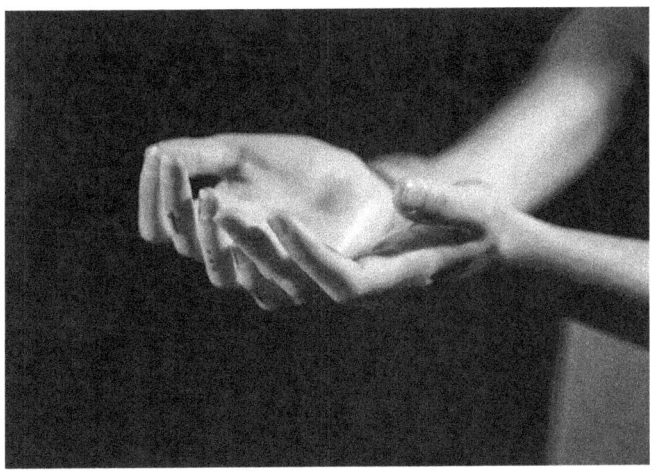

What is Reiki?

Reiki is the art of healing with hands. It appeared in

ancient times, but in the form in which it exists now, it was formed by the Japanese Buddhist Mikao Usui in 1922 and is of great interest to supporters of alternative medicine. Currently, Reiki is a whole system of exposure to the human body with hands.

Reiki is often literally translated as universal life energy. Healing is carried out not by physical methods, but by means of directed energy flow, and at once on several levels - physical, mental and spiritual. Reiki contributes to the healing of the body, eliminates physical fatigue, emotional stress. Reiki energy spiritually cleanses a person, including eliminating addictions, which are often called bad habits. It increases the energy and creative potential of a person, which means that it opens up new opportunities for him.

Reiki is not an artificially created system. It is based on the natural movement, the instinctive direction of energy. Everyone has experience when, having hit something, you immediately put your hand to the sore spot. At the same time, it immediately becomes easier and I want some more time to warm the place of the bruise with the warmth of my hands. In this case, the person himself eases his condition. His hand at this time directs the energy of the body and emotions exactly to the address. Energy effects on the body can also be carried out consciously, developing your abilities and applying certain efforts.

Reiki includes techniques that originated in antiquity - Reiki healers of Tibet practiced many centuries ago. Then this method of energy exposure spread through Egypt, Ancient Greece and Rome to India, China and reached Japan. Mikao Usui only revived and summarized knowledge about the healing effects of the hands.

There is nothing mystical about transmitting energy through the hand. This phenomenon is inherent in nature, in which everything is interconnected and matters. The hand from the point of view of the human energy system, which is itself part of nature, is an energy channel. Therefore, it can give and receive energy. The direction of energy movement depends on the intent of the healer. He can remove the negative from the patient or from his own part of the body, or vice versa, fill it with healthy energy. By practicing Reiki, a person does not create anything new, he only reveals his energy channels, develops intuition, the ability to concentrate, and perceive information from the outside on a subconscious level.

The effect of Reiki occurs by itself, for this, the healer does not need to make any special efforts: he simply enters the Reiki stream and pronounces the necessary affirmation. Then it remains only to direct energy to a specific part of the body or a diseased organ. Healing energy produces a positive result, regardless of how accurately the hands are applied to the sore spot. The healer during the treatment session becomes part of the cosmic energy system, through which this energy is transmitted to the patient.

The Reiki experience is naturally conveyed by the master. Hand healing cannot be taught, like writing or counting. It is an important mood, subtle feeling, inner freedom. If this is inherent in a person and he trusts his intuition, then accepting Reiki will be easy for him.

Reiki affects not only people but also animals, plants. Reiki treatment has no contraindications and side effects. That is why this healing method is of great interest to people who have chronic diseases and want to improve their health, restore physical and mental strength.

Reiki as a healing system has been researched for a long time at the US National Center for Complementary and Alternative Medicine. Scientists have confirmed the safety of this treatment and the absence of side effects from it, although in the process of treatment, uncomfortable conditions may appear (drowsiness, fever, unexpected surge of strength, etc.). The effectiveness of Reiki in the fight against stress, fear, emotional disturbances, mental trauma, and chronic pain has been confirmed. This allows you to use Reiki in chronic diseases, to prepare for surgical interventions, recovery from illness and stress.

Reiki eliminates the energy imbalance in the body, removes energy blocks and restores balance. Everything is simple and effective. Reiki practice does not contradict any religious beliefs and is combined with many traditional and non-traditional methods of treatment - acupressure, massage, psychotherapy, physiotherapy. As a rule, a complex effect on the body is always more effective in treatment. Since Reiki does not have a side effect, it can be used as an adjunct treatment for many diseases. The energy from the hands is perceived by the body through clothes, plaster bandages, etc. since it is all-pervasive and there are no material obstacles for it.

Nor does Reiki adversely affect the one who gives Reiki and helps others to get rid of physical pain, moral feelings and mental suffering. During the healing session, neither the healer nor the patient fall into a trance, do not change their consciousness and worldviews. They only achieve peace, spiritual harmony, unity with nature. They have access to the universal energy flow.

Once accepting initiation from a Reiki mentor, they subsequently use Reiki energy automatically. All adjustments to the space energy system at the right time occur by themselves, without effort and tension.

Why Reiki?

Reiki helps harmonize body and soul. Many diseases develop against the background of prolonged and frequent stresses, psychological problems. Finding peace of mind, solving personal problems and internal harmonization are of great importance for the recovery or prevention of disease. Therefore, Reiki benefits not only patients but also healers.

With the help of Reiki, they awaken the kundalini - vital energy. In esotericism and eastern philosophy, it is represented in the form of a snake, curled up in a ring. It is located in the lower body, at the base of the spine. After removing the energy barriers, kundalini begins to actively circulate along the spine and throughout the body. In Eastern philosophy and medicine, this is given key importance in the light of maintaining health, youth, and longevity.

The awakening of kundalini positively tunes the entire energy system in the human body. It fills not only physical strength but also mental. Kundalini frees consciousness and awakens inner freedom. The potential of kundalini is huge and immeasurable, the activation of this energy causes drastic changes, and it is impossible to resist them. But this is not necessary since the freely circulating energy harmonizes the whole organism and many areas of life.

The human energy system is represented not only by energy channels but also by chakras. It also includes subtle bodies, which are the shell of the physical body. These subtle bodies, the number of which, according to different systems, is from 3 to 7, significantly affect the physical and mental health of a person, protect from negative external energy. If all the energetic thin shells are in good condition, then a person is healthy and feels an integral personality, he is calm and confident in himself, easily resists all troubles, adapts to changing living conditions.

If disturbances occur at any level in the energy system, then this affects the state of health. If they are associated with subtle bodies, then a person becomes especially vulnerable. Therefore, the treatment of diseases with drugs alone is often ineffective. It is necessary to restore the protective shells and the integrity of the entire energy system in the body, then recovery will come. Reiki helps to achieve just that. The energy flow acts immediately on all subtle bodies and restores the body's natural defense. Restoring subtle bodies usually requires a full course of Reiki healing, as one session is not enough.

Reiki energy can work wonders. Hands-on healing is only the first step. A person who has received the second and third steps of reiki can influence the patient at a considerable distance, both on the physical level, and help to correct karma, that is, fate.

REIKI

2 REIKI FUNDAMENTALS

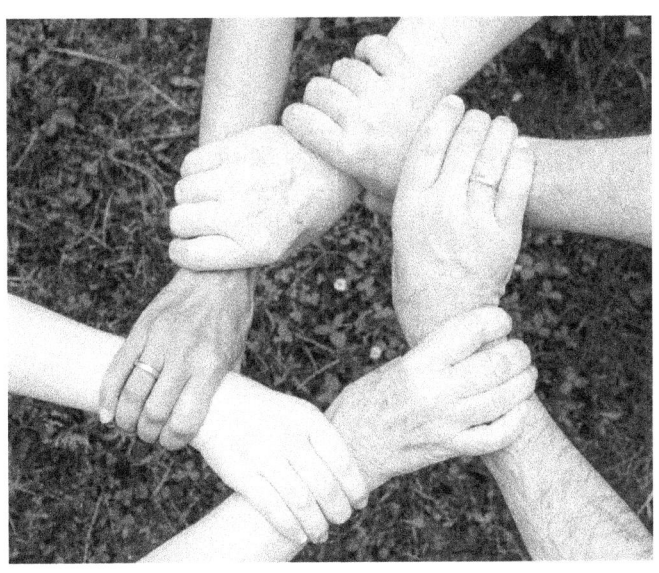

Reiki masters in the Reiki Alliance have developed their own code of ethics. It contains the basic principles followed by Reiki masters.

1. I respect my parents, spouse, and children, their life values and their needs.

2. I value the support that my family provides me with respect to my life path. In the same way, I support my family.

3. For me, the sincerity of my relationship with my family is of great value.

4. I respect my students and patients, their personality and their life values.

5. In relation to my students and patients, I am free from prejudices regarding their age, nationality, religion, culture, sexual orientation and social status.

6. For me, trust in my students and patients is very important and the same attitude towards me on their part.

7. My relationships with students and patients

lack a sexual connotation.

8. I can allow myself other relationships, except professional, with former students or patients only after a certain time.

9. I reserve the right for the student to choose for himself the master he needs, and for the patient - a different form of treatment if necessary.

10. I make sure that my personal judgments do not overlap with the process of training and treatment.

11. The information I hold about my students and patients is strictly confidential.

12. It is very important for me to be in a state of awareness.

13. During the training and treatment process, I am free from drugs and alcohol.

14. I systematically improve my knowledge, skills, and abilities.

15. I really appreciate my capabilities, I know my abilities and limitations.

16. I deeply and sincerely believe in Reiki and my community.

17. I develop in myself such qualities as kindness, love, and honesty.

18. I realize that I cannot control the healing process, I can only learn from him.

19. I respect life.

20. With regard to money, as well as the property of other people, I am honest and decent.

21. For me, professional integrity is important.

22. I respect other healing methods.

23. I respect the healers of other areas.

24. I am responsible for my decisions, actions, and deeds.

25. I recognize that my lifestyle can affect other people.

26. In resolving conflicts, I act quickly and accurately.

Reiki Principles

The basic principles of Reiki, or the rules, were formulated by Mikao Usui. They were based on his own life experience and were extremely important for the healing of the body, soul, and spirit. Dr. Usui noted that there are certain feelings and emotions that interfere with the spiritual development of a person. This is anger, vanity, heartlessness, insincerity, and ingratitude. Mikao Usui wrote down his rules in short sentences.

1. "It is today that you rejoice and live without anger." This principle implies a joyful perception of all components of human life. Joy begins to be projected onto everything around and those around. Then she returns to her source - the man who sent this feeling to the world. Over time, the habit is formed - to wait for a new day with joy. And even if something happens that does not fit into the state of joy and love, this fact must be

perceived positively, that is, also with joy. After all, everything that is being done, everything is aimed at the spiritual growth of a person.

2. "Just today, live without fuss and expect the best." The meaning of this principle is that you need to live in the present, that is, today, here and now, and at the same time expect the best, trusting the life plan of your higher self. It is important not to cling to the past, which cannot be changed, and at the same time, it's time not to worry about the future. Anxiety creates obstacles, barriers. If you remove them, then life will begin to change for the better. Indeed, the belief that only good things begin to happen in life will grow day by day. If something is done that does not meet a person's expectations and does not fit into his concept of "good," this should be taken as another lesson, experience, and level of spiritual growth.

3. "Today, be full of love and warmth for your neighbor and all living things." It should be remembered that all forms of life have a right to exist and constitute a single system of all living things. And in order to be able to show love for all living things, we must learn to love and accept first of all ourselves, our body, and our essence. As a result, others will respond with love and appreciation.

4. "It is today that I honestly earn a living." In order to stay in the natural stream of life, it is necessary to be honest, first of all, to oneself. If you try to gain any advantage through deception, then blocks will appear on the path of spiritual growth, you should always remember this. Similar causes similar, and, cultivating in ourselves honesty, we thereby cause it in others. In addition, the fact of choosing a profession is also important. A person's path of internal development, the awareness of choice, can lead to her

choice. But also, the choice of a profession can be determined by prestige considerations, pressure from parents or relatives. In this case, there are doubts and insecurities.

5. "Today, be grateful to life and thank for the grace received." The Universe is abundant and we must firmly believe that everything we need, we will certainly get. Sending gratitude to the Universe for the benefits received, we re-launch the energy of abundance, which brings success and prosperity. When we enjoy the bright colors of nature, we experience positive emotions, feel part of a whole, abundant world. When we say thanks, it means that we have already received the gift. The sincerity of thanksgiving reduces the time between the request made and its implementation.

In Reiki practice, there are two more important conditions. First: the patient must ask for healing. You should never impose your services. And the second: during the healing session there should be an exchange of energies. This implies the principle of energy recovery, and not necessarily in monetary terms. It can be a certain service, some gift, etc. For Reiki itself, no one has the right to demand anything, it is not someone else's property. And since the healer during the session transfers energy, while his own does not decrease in any way, then it is only a question of reimbursing the time spent by him.

Reiki Symbols and Their Meanings

Symbols in the Reiki system occupy one of the important places. They represent the material embodiment of energy. Many Reiki practitioners compare symbols with notes in music (a note, as you know, is the embodiment of sound). Just as beautiful music pours from under the fingers of a pianist who can read music, so in the hands of a Reiki master, the symbols make Divine energies sound.

Cho Ku Rei

There are four Reiki symbols. The first character is Cho Ku Rei (Fig. 1).

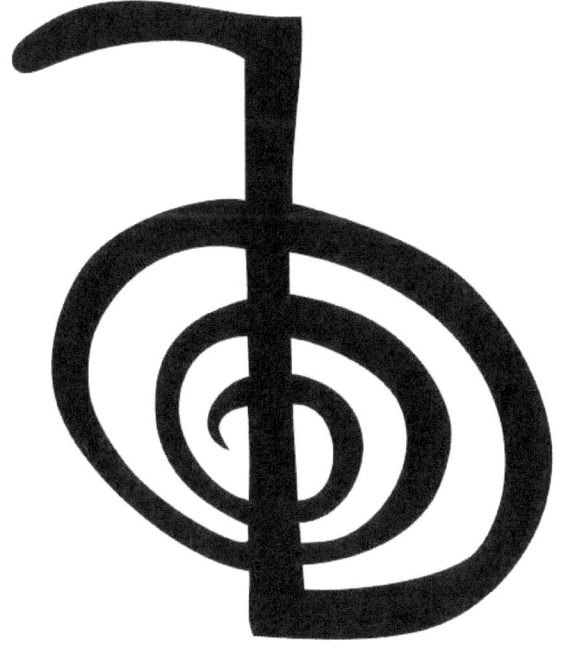

Figure 1. Cho Ku Rei

This symbol has two meanings: "God is here" and "Direct energy to a given point." The main meaning of this symbol is to open access to Reiki energy. Cho Ku

Rei strengthens her flow and healing qualities and creates spiritual protection, weakening the negative effects. In addition, the symbol strengthens intentions, with its help affirmations, become even more powerful. The peculiarity of this basic symbol of Reiki is that it accumulates energy directly at one single point. Cho Ku Rei is used both alone and together with other symbols, possessing the ability to activate them.

Cho Ku Rei helps relieve pain, heal wounds and eliminate nervous irritability. Another purpose of this symbol is to purify the energy space, as well as to fill various objects with energy. It can be household items, crystals, and precious stones, food, medicines, household appliances, indoor plants. It is believed that things will function longer and more successfully, and plants will grow better. This symbol also finds its application when it is necessary to sanctify a place or to initiate (initiation), or in order to develop intuition. In this case, one must meditate on the symbol for 30 minutes twice a day.

The symbol of Cho Ku Rei, the healer mentally draws over his hands before the beginning of the healing session. Then his palms are filled with Reiki energy. The symbol can also be drawn on the surface of the patient's body. At the beginning of the session, this action opens the patient's energy field, and in the end, the transferred energies are strengthened from a universal source. Another way of depicting a symbol is to draw it over the patient's head or at a place that requires treatment. The healer draws Cho Ku Rei with the center of his palm or the "third eye", or he simply visualizes (arises in a mental representation). At the same time, the name of the symbol is pronounced three times in a row.

Sei He Ki

The second character is Sei He Ki (Fig. 2).

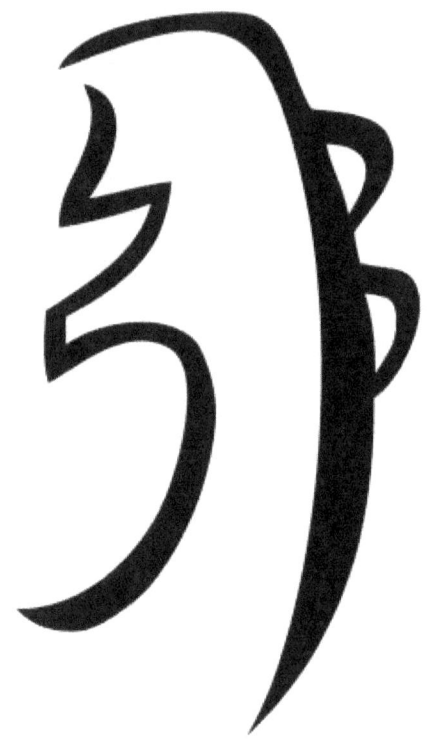

Figure 2. Sei He Ki

It means "The Key to the Absolute", as well as "Man and God merge together." Thus, Sei He Ki symbolizes the harmony of reason and emotions. Like the first character, Sei He Ki protects against any negative. In addition, it is intended to relieve a person of stress, to prevent negative thoughts and emotions from penetrating into his energy field. Finally, Sei He Ki contributes to the awakening of the Divine mind within a person, that is, it changes the reaction of the brain to various life situations. As a result, there is a restoration of harmony and the unity of man with his Higher Self.

Sha Ze Sho Nen

The third symbol is Hon Sha Ze Sho Nen (Fig. 3).

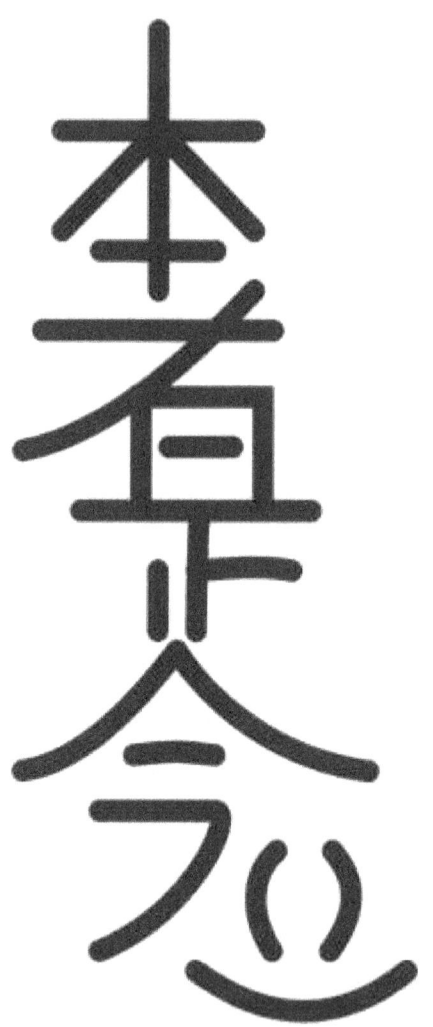

Figure 3. Hon Sha Ze Sho Nen

Each word in this symbol has its own interpretation. Hon: source, origin, land. Sha: "reach the very core of the problem." Ze: "the life-giving center of the universe." Sho: "without time, timeless present." If the first symbol (Cho Ku Rei) is able to focus energy at only one point, then this symbol simultaneously directs the energy flow to several points, as well as from one place on the human body to another. In addition, this symbol transports energy through time and space, that is, the energy flow reaches an event or specific people, both in the present and in the past and future. This is possible due to the fact that Hon Sha Ze Sho Nen symbolizes the concept of "now", excluding the concepts of "past" and "future", they simply do not exist. It is worth realizing it - and ordinary ideas of time break down. True real life is coming, the meaning of which is in the words: "there is no past, present, and future since all this is now." Another meaning of this symbol is in the words: "The Buddha in me unites with the Buddha in you in order to achieve enlightenment and peace." With the help of this symbol, it becomes possible to carry out treatment at a distance, concentrate on what is happening at the moment and bring the person's energy centers into a balanced state.

Dai Ko Myo

The fourth symbol (symbol of the master) is Dai Ko Myo (Fig. 4).

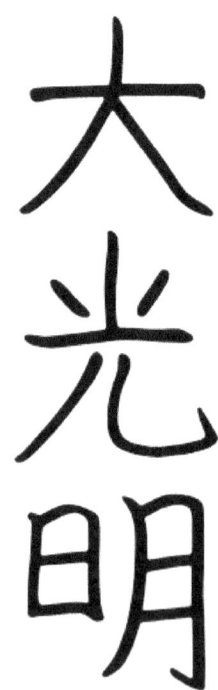

Figure 4. Dai Ko Myo

This is a symbol of the trinity - love, light, and harmony. It is identical to the Christian concept of the Father, the Son, and the Holy Spirit. Strictly speaking, this is not just a symbol, but a certain step towards pure, absolute energy. Dai Ko Myo already contains the three previous characters, so you can use it instead. But in order to master it, it takes time for understanding and awareness. Dai Ko Myo is a symbol of the third stage. Its meaning is contained in the words "Great Shining Light."

There are slight differences in how different Reiki masters draw symbols for their students. In addition, one master could draw the same characters in different ways.

The listed characters are communicated to students during the initiation ritual (or customization, input). Then they gain their strength and effectiveness. First, the master shows the characters to the students and gives them time for them to remember. Symbols penetrate into the energy centers of the student's body and the initiate holds them in his memory so that he can subsequently pass them on (drawing them in front of each new initiate). As already noted, symbols can be activated using visualization, pronouncing their names, using the sketch of the palm. You can just think about the energy of the symbol - and access to this energy will be open.

How Do You Like The Book So Far?

Leave a review on amazon!

If you're undecided, just leave a review later...

Before You Continue… Do You Want to Receive My FREE Bonus that will help to improve your days?

Receive my little small gift for you, just click here
arianaweber.com or write it on web

REIKI

3 YOUR PSYCHIC GIFTS

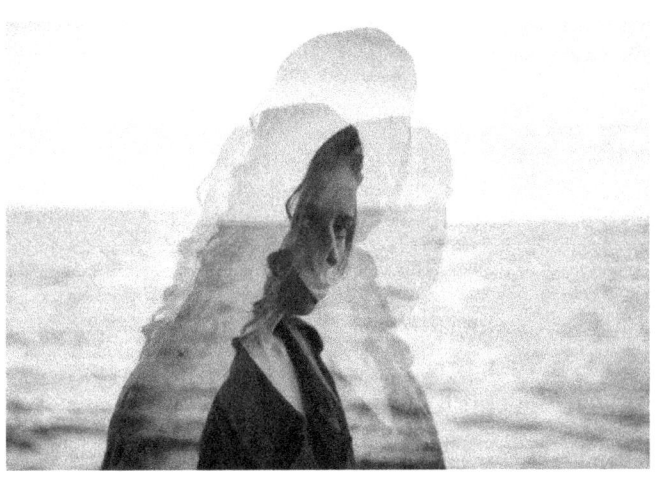

Teaching Reiki

Dr. Usui's Reiki System has two steps. At the first

stage, a person starting to practice Reiki (opens Reiki channels). In the second stage, he is already able to heal (sometimes at a distance, too). In some schools, there are additional or intermediate levels (levels).

As a rule, classes in the first and second steps are held in the form of seminars. These may be seminars of the so-called "weekend" (Saturday - Sunday), or evening courses during the week. Each Reiki teacher builds his seminars individually, but the following points are surely reflected in them: the story of how Dr. Usui rediscovered this ancient teaching in the 20th century; the development of Reiki in the last century (XX century) and at present; information on how this universal vital energy acts; the main positions of the hands are shown. Most importantly, at the first stage, Reiki channels are opened and the students (or initiation) settings.

On the first day of the first-stage workshop, the teacher shows several relaxation exercises - in order to increase perception. After the exercises, the teacher begins to open Reiki channels to the students. So, the first two settings are implemented. The ritual itself, or rite of passage, is as follows:

The student closes his eyes so as not to be distracted, but to concentrate on himself, on his feelings. After that, the teacher sends him a stream of energy, which, reaching the energy centers of the initiate's body, opens Reiki channels. All four Reiki symbols are involved in this action. At the same time, the opening of the four upper chakras takes place - according to the number of settings carried out in the first step. When the first adjustment is made, the heart chakra opens; during the second - the throat center. The third setting affects the frontal chakra and the fourth - on the crown or parietal center. This changes the quality of the chakras.

The phenomenon of settings is that the Reiki channels that are open during settings remain that way forever. Even if a person then does not continue to practice Reiki, his channels are open and can receive and transmit energy. Another feature: since Reiki is an inexhaustible source, the person transmitting Reiki energy does not lose his own and, in addition, the channels of both the transmitter and the receiver are protected from negative energy.

During the opening of the channels, many students have a joyful, positive feeling and pleasant sensations in the body. This, for example, is warmth, or a slight tingling, or trembling. Most of all, these phenomena are felt in the hands - because now it is through them that Reiki energy flows. Many experience a state of enthusiasm, "cordiality" and emotional openness. Next, there is a study of certain positions of the hands, special exercises are performed to develop sensitivity. In the first step, students can already start self-healing and heal other members of the group, but these are only the first steps. After passing the first stage, it is important to transfer Reiki energy as often as possible. The improvement of its course directly depends on the frequency of its transmission. In this sense, Reiki is a gift, and for the one who gives it, too. And of course, the aspect of personal growth does not stand aside. After opening channels and the practice of energy transfer, the previously hidden sides of the personality of a positive plan are manifested.

2-3 months after passing the first stage, you can start training at the second stage of Reiki. This is the optimal gap between the steps, although, with daily practice, Reiki can reduce the break to three weeks. However, the main thing here is not the calendar dates, but the inner need of the person. This may be the desire to improve, and the desire to spread Reiki, that is, follow Reiki-do ("do" means "way"). In any case, it will be best if a person listens to himself, trusts his intuition and, if necessary, gives himself time to "mature" to go to the next level.

In the second stage, settings are also made - the opening of new energy channels takes place, and they, like the channels opened in the first stage, remain effective for life. Immediately after the settings, students learn the spelling and names (mantras) of the first three Reiki symbols. At the first stage, these symbols were not yet known to the students; only the teacher used them to open the channels. Now, students are given time to study them visually (you can't write them down) and permanently capture them in their memory. After this, the students begin to do exercises on the use of symbols. It should be emphasized that despite the fact that outwardly the second-stage seminars are very similar to the first-level seminars, there is a qualitative difference between them. After all, all students who have passed to the second level have already practiced how to deal with Reiki energy.

The second stage is more saturated and more intense than the first since the energy of Reiki is now emitted not only by the hands (as in the first stage) but also by the crown center (chakra in the region of the crown of the head). Pupils master the ability to focus energy, as well as transmit it to a distance. The latter seems fantastic, however, for Reiki energy, there are no time or spatial boundaries. And everyone who is engaged in the second stage can be convinced of it. Finally, the time required for healing is significantly reduced. If at the first stage this required about 1.5 hours, then the second healing session lasts 10-15 minutes. Often, the healer himself (a practicing student) feels how his body transfers vital energy.

The third step is called the workshop. As the name implies, at this stage initiation into a Reiki master takes place. People come to her who decided to devote themselves completely to Reiki, who realized that Reiki is their way. The third step in form is not a copy of the first and second. First of all, he who decides to become a Reiki master is looking for a teacher. The fundamental point here is the full confidence of both the student and the master. A prerequisite for training at the third level - you must have at least 1-year experience in the second stage program.

First, the student assists in the workshops of his master. This is an important moment of training at the third stage when the future master's own ideas are formed. They may conflict with the views of the teacher. Often at this stage, there is a crisis in the relationship between student and teacher. If it is successfully overcome, the actual training of the future master comes. It takes several days. The student is given the master symbol of Dai Ko Myo and the third stage is set up. Then there is the practice of conducting seminars of the first and second stages, i.e., first all of their stages are thoroughly passed (more precisely, they are repeated - after all, the future master once passed them himself), then the student becomes a master.

It is interesting to note that if in other practices (yoga, qigong, tai chi) the idea of the universality of the Universe does not arise immediately, but in stages, then in Reiki, this happens already at the very beginning of training. In addition, it does not take many years to devote to mastering special exercises.

The one who has completed the third stage greatly increases the possibility of receiving and transmitting energy. In addition, the spiritual aspect is also greatly increasing - the former student is now able to lead others along the Reiki path. Setting up the master stage allows you to carry out all the settings of the previous stages extremely unusually. There is a feeling of belonging to the Higher power. An important condition for the past third step is the obligatory work with students. Pupils are the mirror of the master, they give him the opportunity to better understand himself and, as a result, to advance more successfully along the path of self-knowledge. The third stage ends with the title of master, and he enters the path of life-long Reiki.

After each step, the so-called periods of "purification" begin in psychological terms. At this time, thoughts and feelings that did not give rest for a long time, for example, old resentments, may come back. Fears may arise. However, the cleansing phase is also characterized by positive aspects. So, some may quit smoking, and this happens completely painlessly; there is no hunger when a person fasts. Thus, the period of purification gives a chance to acquire good habits and get rid of bad ones.

Opportunities – Reiki and the Path to Enlightenment

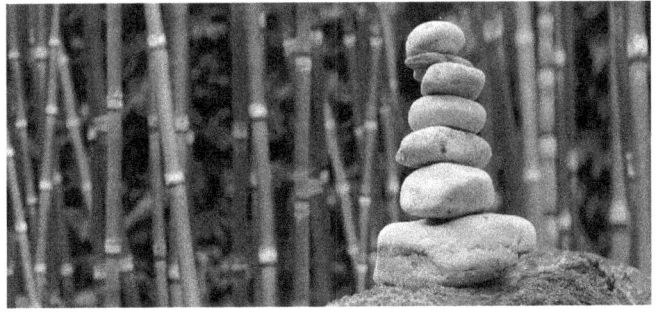

Since Reiki is that universal life energy that permeates all living things, it also has a healing effect on animals and plants. At the heart of the healing (treatment) of animals lies the same system as in the treatment of people. This coincidence is not accidental: after all, the chakras of the representatives of the fauna are mainly in the same place as in humans. What is also important: animals feel better Reiki energy and do not oppose its adoption. And in this sense, their treatment is sometimes more effective. It is only important to remember that if certain symptoms of the disease are present, you need to contact your veterinarian for help as soon as possible and only then apply Reiki. In this case, Reiki will support the treatment of animals.

Reiki cannot only heal pets (as well as wild ones) but also supports the well-being of healthy people. It has been observed that animals like to accept Reiki energy. For a Reiki practitioner, such feedback is extremely important. By the behavior of the animal, the healer sees how accurate his actions are.

Plants are even more sensitive to energy. And this is not surprising: because they live due to the fact that they feed on the energy of the sun and are the green lungs of our planet. In plants, the ability to transfer energy was originally laid down. But sometimes the plants themselves need healing. This applies to sick indoor plants, and garden plants, and trees in the forest. If you regularly direct the energy of Reiki to the roots of plants, then the result will not slow down. You can also conduct such an experiment: pick up a handful of grains and direct Reiki energy to them, and then plant them in the ground. Grains processed in this way will have a much higher growth rate than untreated grains.

Surprisingly, it is a fact: Reiki affects not only wildlife but also on inanimate objects. For example, with Reiki energy, you can charge the battery, it is easier to sharpen the knife, make the fabric more durable. This is understandable if we adhere to the point of view that everything in the Universe is alive, everything is animated, and if the Universe itself lives, then to a certain extent the line between the living and nonliving disappears.

So, if you transfer Reiki energy to a discharged battery, it will recharge (that is, the remaining energy in it will be activated). However, the second time it will not be able to charge it. Similarly, you can make a car work if it has a stalled motor, or fix a door lock that is stuck. A stopped clock will also work if you direct Reiki energy to it. The crystal can be charged with this energy, and then it will radiate Reiki. Some master's use charged crystals as a talisman. With the help of Reiki energy, you can harmonize your home, paying special attention to the bedroom and corners during this action (they are especially vulnerable to the penetration of negative energy). But in this case, it is necessary to pass the second and third steps, all four symbols of Reiki are involved here.

Reiki energy can be invaluable in critical health and life conditions. However, it should be remembered that the transfer of Reiki energy does not replace qualified medical care. Therefore, you must first call a doctor. After his intervention, the use of Reiki accelerates the healing process. It is important to know the following: if a fracture occurs, first you need to perform all the necessary medical actions (apply gypsum, etc.). Impossible to apply Reiki immediately, otherwise the bones may not grow together correctly. If a person has an open wound, it must first be disinfected, and then Reiki should be passed, and hands should be kept at a distance of 3-5 cm from the wound. Reiki provides effective assistance in the event of an insect bite. If you transfer the energy of Reiki for 20 minutes, the poison is neutralized. During a heart attack, immediately after a doctor's call (before his arrival), it is necessary to transfer Reiki (this is important!) to the parietal chakra. Reiki also helps in a state of shock. The transmitting energy at the same time supports the conversation with the victim.

The possibilities of Reiki are manifested in two other important aspects of being - the emergence of a new life and the process of death, dying. As a rule, the last topic for almost all people is largely painful. Perhaps here one should not even speak about death itself, but about fear of it. However, in all religions it is emphasized that death is not the end of life, it means the beginning of a new existence but already modified. Therefore, it would be more correct to designate the fear of death as the fear of "nothing." And this fear arises at the subconscious level, that is, in that area that is not realized by a person and is not controlled by him.

However, in contrast to irrational fear, which is the fear of death, there is a rational fear. This is a fear of the disease. As you know, Reiki can heal even in severe cases. Therefore, the fear of the disease is overcome. And just as Reiki can overcome fear of disease, fear of death is also overcome through this universal art. The German philosopher Arthur Schopenhauer (1788-1860) absolutely justifiably said that if people are so afraid that they will cease to exist after death, then it is worth remembering that they did not exist in the same way before their birth, that is before they were born.

A person practicing Reiki is filled with vital energy, he realizes that since he receives this energy from the Universe, the Universe is also filled with the energy of joy and love. And in this sense, death is a transformation of life in the same cycle of inexhaustible life energy. Of course, for those who say goodbye to life, and for those whom he leaves, such experiences are not an easy process. Reiki art can help you survive this moment. Reiki practitioners who surround the dying person are able to convey to him the feeling of the positive changes that have occurred to them under the influence of Reiki.

No less important is the influence of Reiki at the time of the birth of a future life. During pregnancy, Reiki protects the unborn baby from diseases and other negative influences. Efficiency increases if Reiki is transmitted not only by the expectant mother but also by the father. Reiki also supports the woman who is carrying a child, for example, contributes to the disappearance of nausea. In the fourth month of pregnancy, when a growing baby already hears the voices of their future parents, the emotional connection between them can be strengthened with the help of Reiki. It is important to pass the Reiki to the child before his sleep and awakening.

During childbirth, Reiki energy helps to alleviate pain. It is possible at this moment to transfer Reiki directly to the crown chakra. The best option is if immediately after birth the father takes the baby in his arms and hands him the Reiki (the mother herself is not able to do this). The energy of Reiki is no less important during infancy, since in the first year of life when the foundations of the child's relationship with the world are laid: fear and doubt or joy and trust. Receiving Reiki from parents, the child is convinced that the world in which Reiki flows is safe. Reiki received by the child contributes to his physical and spiritual development. If everything is fine from the first steps in life, this is a favorable start in life.

Another of the possibilities of Reiki is that this art is harmoniously combined with other methods of treatment, for example, with traditional medicine. If a person has broken a leg or arm, then they will put gypsum on him and leave the broken limb alone. The very restoration of functions lost due to trauma is possible with the flow of vital energy. Reiki strengthens this.

Reiki also complements and enhances the effect of massage, whether classic or Japanese (shiatsu). In the first case, Reiki helps eliminate deeply hidden energy blocks. In addition, it should be borne in mind that the massage therapist, when conducting a session, is exposed to the negative energy that accompanies the patient's illness. Reiki just protects the specialist from such an impact. Finally, if a massage therapist practices Reiki, he can more accurately determine the location of energy blocks (due to the fact that he has increased susceptibility to the flow of energy) and remove them.

Shiatsu massage differs from the usual one in that it is performed with fingers only and not with the whole hand. And the purpose of this method is somewhat different from classic massage. In shiatsu, the focus is on points that are located on the energy paths. By pressing on them, the energy flow is increased and blockades (blocks) are lifted. If during the shiatsu session you pass the Reiki, the unlocking of the energy paths will be faster and easier.

Reiki is very well combined with such non-traditional methods of medicine as homeopathy, flower therapy, and aromatherapy. Homeopathy (founded by Samuel Hahnemann in 1810) is based on the principle that "the like is cured by the like". In other words, the substance that caused the disease, in small doses, can cure it. When diluting or grinding the substance, its medicinal effect is enhanced. At the heart of homeopathy is the energy effect, so Reiki combines very well with homeopathy. Reiki can be used in the preparation of various homeopathic medicines, or you can charge already prepared ones.

It is proved that Reiki art has such a unique ability that it can heal a person from his photograph, by talking to him on the phone, if the healer has personal belongings of the person, as well as if the acquaintances or friends of the patient are intermediaries.

Flower therapy by the English physician Edward Bach (1886–1936) is based on the effects of the energy of flowers, herbs, and trees. As you know, bodily diseases are preceded by spiritual problems caused by feelings such as anger, fear, resentment, hatred, etc. It has long been noticed that certain plants help in such conditions. For example, in overcoming fears, aspen, cherry plum, red chestnut, mountain rose are effective. Wild apple, elm, larch, oak, pine, sweet chestnut help to overcome despair. The vital energy of these and other plants is placed in the essence. Reiki will help to strengthen the effect of essences and if you use it in the cooking process, and if you process energy ready-made essences with Reiki.

In recent decades, interest in aromatherapy has increased. Aromatherapy is a treatment method using natural essential oils that are introduced into the body through the respiratory tract, skin and mucous membranes. The term "aromatherapy" was proposed by the French chemist Rene Maurice Gattfosse in the early twentieth century. When he burned his hand and lowered it into a vessel with lavender oil, he found that the burn healed much faster and did not leave scars. He outlined his observations of the properties of essential oils in the book Aromatherapy.

However, mankind has been familiar with essential oils for over 6 thousand years. In ancient Egypt, China, Persia, and India, essential oils were used in almost all areas of life. Essential oils have healing and cleansing properties and unique aromas. They help to find peace of mind lost in our lives and heal bodily diseases. Reiki enhances the healing effects of essential oils.

It is possible to process Reiki energy not only with essential oils but also with spices. They, like essential oils, have been known to man for many thousands of years and are more gentle ways of influencing the body than chemicals (medicines). Spices are known to affect digestion and blood circulation. It is no secret that at present in spices, as in other products, particles of harmful substances that penetrate from soil, air, water are contained. If you direct the energy of Reiki to spices, then the effect of heavy metals, pesticides, etc. is neutralized.

The possibilities of Reiki are well manifested in Reiki groups, which consist of 2-8 people. This is especially useful for those people who have chronic diseases. In this case, the regular transfer and reception of Reiki energy in Reiki groups helps to improve the condition. In a Reiki group, each of its members is both a healer and a receiver of healing. A session of taking Reiki energy takes on average about 15 minutes per participant (sometimes Reiki energy can be transmitted longer if necessary).

Reiki energy transfer is possible not only in groups of

more than two people but with your partner. If everyone in the pair has passed the first stage, this will be enough to give the relationship a much greater depth and harmony, as well as improve each other's health. A good opportunity for this is shared meditation. To carry it out, you need to sit opposite each other, raise both hands to chest level. In this case, the palm of the right hand looks down, and the palm of the left is turned up. After that, you should put your palms in the palms of your partner, close your eyes and direct the flow of energy to the partner, and then strengthen its movement in the opposite direction - from the partner to yourself. This should be repeated several times. This cycle will greatly enhance the Reiki energy that circulates within each of the partners.

The possibilities of Reiki are not limited to those described above. There is one more amazing property: in addition to the settings that the master performs at the seminars, there is also a correspondence or independent setting. Currently, it has become possible for two reasons. Firstly, due to the existence of morphogenetic fields. This theory was proposed by the

Russian scientist Alexander Gurvich in 1922, and in the 70s of the twentieth century was developed in the works of a biologist from England Rupert Sheldrake. Its essence lies in the fact that the formation of living organisms and inanimate structures are influenced by morphogenetic fields that are transmitted through the temporal and spatial aspects. In this regard, the formation of organisms is more active, as well as certain changes in the behavior of people and animals. In practice, this means that if in a certain region of the Earth an animal species adopts, for example, a new manner of behavior, then such behavior in animals of the same species is observed almost everywhere. In addition, it is easier to digest. Experiments on rats confirmed this fact.

It was noted that during the settings, Reiki masters also formed a morphogenetic field. And since lately the Reiki teachings have expanded significantly and gained many supporters and followers, it has become much easier to make settings. In this regard, it became possible to make settings remotely (at a distance, it is done by the master) and independently. Naturally, tuning yourself is more difficult. It is preceded by a two-week preparation (30 minutes per day), which distinguishes it from the setting carried out directly by the master.

So, first of all, breathing exercises are necessary to carry out the adjustment yourself. This fact has its justification. Life energy can be obtained in two ways: through Reiki channels (who have them open) and through breathing.

REIKI

4 SAFE PSYCHIC DEVELOPMENT

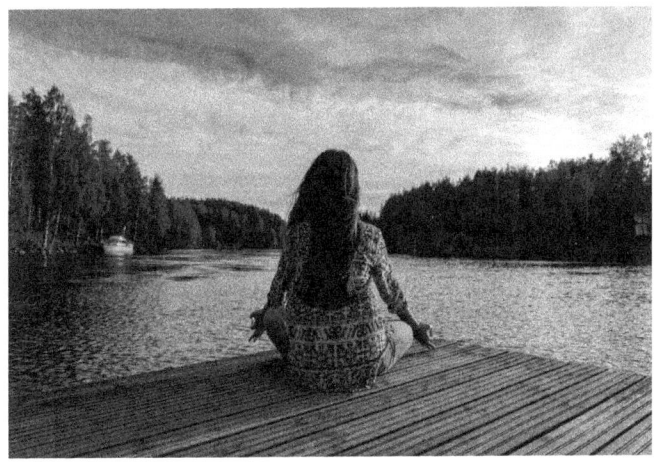

As noted, you will most probably need hands-on from a teacher to open your Reiki channels. However, this is not all. The life energy is also obtained through breathing. This could also open up the Reiki channels. In any case, whether you have your Reiki channels open fully, a little, or not at all, the following exercises are sure going to take you several steps further.

Basic Breathing Exercise

1. Place your left hand over your right and place both hands on your stomach.

2. Take three deep breaths (while inhaling the stomach a little stuck out) and exhale. Feel the pleasant warmth pouring inside the abdomen. The abdomen is the sacred chakra, or svadhisthana, which transfers very strong energy and charges the chakras of the hands.

3. Place the right hand over the left and put both hands in the middle of the chest - this is the place of the heart chakra (anahata). Sensations can be different: warmth, or trembling in the hands, or the appearance of joy. Holding your hands in the middle of the chakra, take a few breaths.

4. Reposition the left hand over the right, put your hands on the sacred chakra (stomach), take three deep breaths and exhale, that is, charge the chakras of the hands.

5. Put your hands on the throat chakra (vishudha) area almost under the larynx. In this case, the fingers are located on the cervical vertebrae and the palms of the larynx.

6. Charge the hand chakras again as described above.

7. Fold your hands in the shape of a "bucket". Bring your hands to the frontal chakra (ajna) - this is the place between the eyebrows, the so-called "third eye", and keep them at a distance of 3 cm from it. Focus on your feelings.

8. Recharge the chakras of the hands.

9. Bring your hands to the crown chakra (sahasrara). Arrange your hands so that they touch the chakra only with your fingertips. In this area, the energy flux may be somewhat

smaller.

Breathing techniques allow the practitioner to control the energy in his body. Proper distribution of energy in the body contributes to a significant improvement in health, both physical and psycho-emotional.

Controlled Breathing Exercise

1. Its main purpose is to remove all blockages that impede the flow of energy.

1. Sit on a chair or on the floor. It is important to keep your back straight, but not to strain, hands should be relaxed, as if hanging down.

2. Take a deep breath and focus on the chakras of the hands - this is the middle of the palms.

3. At the next inhalation, slowly raise your hands to chest level and at the end of this movement, complete the inspiration. Attention is still paid to the chakras of the hands. Turning your

hands with your palms down, exhale and slowly lower your hands again. Focus on exhaling, feeling the chakras of the hands "breathe" (in the process of lowering them). Before repeating this fragment of the exercise, the arms hang again, relaxed, breathing is normal. Repeat a fragment - from three to five times. If warmth or some vibration is felt when performing movements, this means that energy is flowing.

4. Next is the study of the four upper chakras. First hearty. After taking a breath, you need to focus on this center and slowly raise your hands up. Turning the palms down, exhale and direct energy to the heart chakra. Repeat this movement three to five times. Each time, the flow of energy becomes freer, heat spreads in the chest area.

5. Take a breath, focus on the throat chakra, and slowly raise your hands up. Turn your hands with your palms down, exhale and direct energy to the throat chakra. Repeat this

fragment 3-5 times.

6. Inhale, pay all attention to the frontal chakra. Slowly raise your hands up. Turning your hands with your palms down, exhale and direct energy to the area of the frontal chakra. Repeat three to five times.

7. Take a breath, focus on the crown chakra. Slowly raise your hands up. Turn your hands with your palms down, exhale and direct energy to the crown chakra. So do 3-5 times. In this exercise, coordination of breathing and hand movements is very important: inhalation - all attention to the chakra; exhale - energy is sent to the chakra. The described movements should be done at an average pace (they take from 15 to 20 minutes) twice a day in the sequence shown.

Visualization Exercise

1. Take a comfortable pose (sitting, standing or lying). Close your eyes and relax. Breathing is

free.

2. Present a luminous white ball above your head in the area of the crown chakra. Take a breath, and as you exhale imagine that energy is added in a white ball and its radiance is enhanced. Next, visualize how light from the ball flows into the crown chakra. Alternate inhalations and exhalations and imagine that with each breath in the chakra comes pure life energy, and with each breath, there is a release from the energy of the "contaminated", expended.

3. Mentally slowly lower the ball to the frontal chakra and imagine that the glow of the ball becomes purple. Take inspiration and exhalation again, getting rid of the spent energy and absorbing clean energy.

4. Lower the ball to the level of the throat chakra. The glow of purple should turn blue. Often at this level, a sensation of warmth occurs, and the color changes its shades according to inhalations and exhalations:

inhalation - the color becomes more saturated, exhalation - the thickening of the color is replaced by transparency.

5. Lower the ball to the area of the heart chakra. The blue color of the ball transforms into emerald green. With each exhalation, the color darkens, with each breath it brightens.

6. Mentally take the ball with both hands (the ball again acquired a dazzling white color, as at the very beginning of the exercise). When inhaling, direct its glow to your hands, while exhaling, the energy from the hands again rushes into the ball.

7. Relax, rest and repeat all the stages of the exercise again.

There are situations in which all the human chakras are in close contact with each other and energy is exchanged between them. This, for example, occurs when a person assumes a fetal position. Accordingly, in the fetus in the womb, the chakras are adjacent to each other.

When you perform this exercise for the first time, fatigue may appear, then you should pause and only after that start a repetition. This exercise must be performed at least twice daily. As a result, there should come a state in which a luminous ball appears in the imagination by itself and in the same way, without any effort, the color of each of the chakras changes. If this condition lasts about two weeks, you can continue to the next exercise. This exercise increases the energy of the chakras.

Exercise "Meditation at a Light Point"

This exercise has some analogies to the previous exercise. And it also involves the energy of light. But if in the exercise described above, the energy was concentrated in the ball, then in "Meditation" it focuses on a dazzling bright point. This exercise is best done before bedtime.

1. Close your eyes, relax. Consider what appears before the inner eye. It can be some specific images or some dark mass.

2. Imagine a point of some color, focus on it and begin to reduce this point in size.

3. Imagine how this point, reduced to almost microscopic dimensions, "takes off."

This exercise should be completed within a few weeks. At first, it's important to simply visualize the light point, not paying attention to its color. In the future, when this is achieved, it should focus on its presentation of emerald green, blue, purple and white colors (it is necessary to observe just such a sequence). As a result, the ability to alternately visualize all these colors should appear in a few seconds. Such a trained ability is an indicator that all barriers are removed in the mind.

After mastering the previous exercises and meditation at the light point, you can proceed to self-tuning. But first, you need to remember the names and images (how they look) of the four characters, with which you can independently open the Reiki channel.

Reiki Self-Tuning

1. The whole process of self-tuning is as follows.

1. Create a calm atmosphere, come in a pleasant mood and meditate on a light point.

2. Without opening your eyes, lay your hands on the heart chakra and recite the mantra "yinya no ay" aloud. Visualize the first symbol. Next, imagine a green dot of light. At this point, the opening of the heart chakra will occur.

3. Transfer hands from the heart chakra to the throat. Say the mantra "yinya no chi" and visualize the second symbol. After that, visualize the light point in blue. With its activation, the throat chakra will open.

4. Next is the opening of the frontal chakra. To do this, put your hands on the frontal chakra, pronounce the mantra "yinya no ki" and

visualize the symbol "three" and the light point in purple. The frontal chakra is open, now it remains to open the last, crown, chakra.

5. Put your hands on the area of the crown chakra, pronounce the mantra "yinya no itchi" and present the symbol "four", then visualize a white dot. Now there is a connection between all open chakras. Reiki channel is open, it allows the flow of Reiki energy. In the following days, it is necessary to practice the transmission and reception of Reiki energy.

Enhance Your Reiki Tuning with a Specialized Diet

Before carrying out self-tuning (as, however, and before full-time tuning by the master), you can follow a certain diet, or you can do without it. There are no strict rules in this regard. It is much more important to have the appropriate emotional attitude. If there is a desire to eat in a certain way before setting up, we give an approximate composition of the diet.

On the first day of the diet, it is recommended to drink only water, not to do heavy physical work and to remain more relaxed. On the second day, eat fruit and drink fruit juices (preferably apple, pear, and grape). On the third day, vegetables and cheese are added to the fruit diet and juices. You can also eat yogurt and drink sugar-free fruit tea. On the fourth day of special nutrition, cheese and eggs should be excluded from the diet. It is allowed to drink milk, juices, eat fruits and any vegetarian food. On the fifth, sixth and seventh days continue to eat vegetarian dishes and fruits. Avoid flour, tea, and coffee. In the following days, you can return to normal food, but this should be done gradually. The diet helps to cleanse the body so that it becomes more susceptible to tuning.

REIKI

5 SPIRITUAL PERFECTION AND REIKI

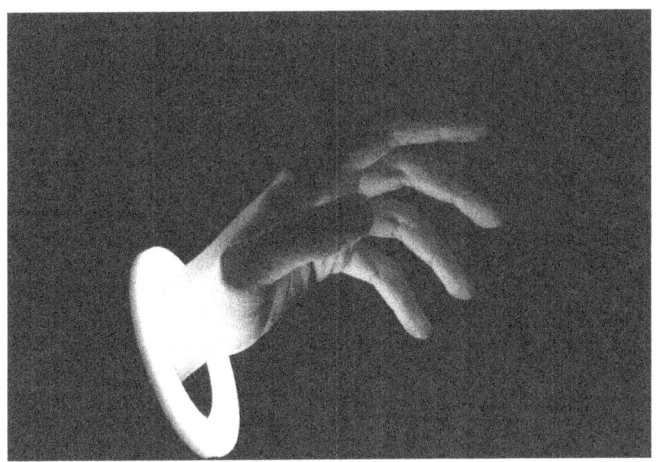

God turns his words to everyone, but not everyone hears. But he who seeks will find sooner or later, and everyone will be rewarded according to his desires. When practicing Reiki, I realized that all the great religions aspire to the same goal. This conclusion suggests itself, there is only one Truth, or Reality, although it can be interpreted and implemented in different ways at different levels.

Externally, the attributes of world religions may differ. However, a comparative analysis of the acts and commandments of the great saints and ascetics of different faiths proves the commonality of their goals and theological approaches. It should be noted that modern science is gradually departing from the positions of militant materialism.

At the beginning of the 20th century, Einstein's theory of relativity shocked the foundations of traditional ideas about the universe. For the first time in academic circles, the idea was voiced that space and time are not absolute, but relative and mass and energy pass into each other. Even earlier, in 1801, the result of a simple but historically important experiment by Thomas Young on the passage of sunlight through two vertical slits made scientists think about the presence of consciousness in photons!

Max Planck discovered that energy is not radiated directionally, but in portions of particles called quanta. Louis de Broglie shocked his contemporaries, suggesting that not only the waves are composed of particles, but also the particles have a wave nature. Subsequently, he turned out to be right, and this concept is now known as the "Bohr principle of correspondence." Heisenberg completed the destruction of the mechanistic view of the world, discovering the law of the ratio of uncertainties. The uncertainty of the atomic energy suggests the absence of objective reality as such.

These and other exciting discoveries led scientists to reconsider the deterministic, mechanistic view of matter. A new view of things is surprisingly similar to what has long been proposed by many mystics and spiritual teachers.

I will cite the often-quoted statement by Sir James Jeans: "The universe more and more resembles a great thought, not a giant mechanism. The mind no longer looks like an uninvited guest of the universe. We are beginning to suspect that he should be welcomed as the creator and ruler of the material world."

For millennia, man has sought answers to questions about the origin and purpose of the conscious principle. The following quote reflects the similar aspirations of human thought: "A man is a part of the whole, which we call the Universe, a part limited in time and space. He feels himself, his thoughts and feelings as something independent and unique, which is a kind of optical illusion. Such a mistake makes us live in an illusory world of our own desires and limit ourselves to communication with a narrow circle of people close to us. Our task is to overcome the inertness of thinking and embrace the whole world, in all its greatness and splendor." These words do not belong to the mystic, not to the spiritual master, as you might think, but to Albert Einstein.

The Reiki system offers effective ways of self-realization of consciousness and gives answers about its origin and purpose. The ultimate goal of Reiki art is to achieve spiritual perfection by people of any faith, including atheists.

All the great world religions can be considered on two levels: popular, ritual-ostentatious and at the highest, religious and philosophical. Most ordinary people perceive religion at the ritualistic level and are usually ignorant of its philosophy. Due to historical, geographical, cultural, linguistic, intellectual and other factors, world religions clearly differ at the level of ritual-cult attributes. But, studying the religious and philosophical concepts of different faiths and the teachings of the great prophets, it is easy to find that they have much in common.

I would like to show you the goals and methods of the great world religions in the form in which the greatest teachers preach.

Hinduism - the Union of the Atman with Brahman

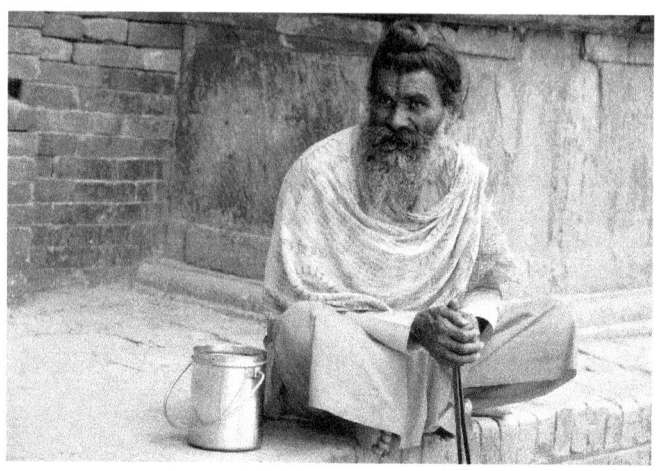

At the ritualistic level in Hinduism, there are no gods and goddesses, but at the philosophical level, they are all manifestations of one supreme deity called Brahman. The following is a passage from the Upanishads, the holy book of the Hindus.

"Before creation, Brahman existed without manifesting himself. From the unmanifest, he created manifestation. He made himself out of himself. Therefore, it exists by itself."

In the Bhagavad Gita, Brahman says through the

mouth of Sri Krishna: "People whose insight has been dulled by worldly passions, have established a particular ritual or cult and turn to various deities under the influence of their innate drives. But it doesn't matter which deity the believer chooses to worship. If he has faith, I make her unshakable. Endowed with the faith I sent, he worships this deity and receives from him everything he prays for. In reality, only I give."

Brahman is manifested in every being as Atman. "I am the Atman that dwells in the soul of every mortal being. I am the beginning, life itself and the end of everything."

Believers can achieve Brahman in many ways, but the best of them is meditation. In the sutras of Patanjali Yoga, we read: "The form of worship, which consists in contemplating Brahman, surpasses ritual worship with material sacrifices."

One way to achieve God, or Brahman, is yoga, which means union with God. Although it is very intensively used by Indians for spiritual development, in reality, yoga is not religious in nature. People of various faiths can use it to their advantage.

There are many types of yoga: hatha yoga, bhakti yoga, mantra yoga, yantra yoga, raja yoga, etc. Raja yoga is considered the highest and teaches the knowledge of God through meditation. Patanjali, the father of yoga, distinguishes eight stages of perfection.

1. **Pit** - abstinence from evil deeds.
2. **Niyama** - the observance of purity, chastity, discipline, reflection, and dedication to God.
3. **Asana** - a static pose.
4. **Pranayama** - breath control.
5. **Pratyahara** - the direction of consciousness inward.
6. **Dharana** - concentration.
7. **Dhyana** - meditation (contemplation).
8. **Samadhi** - enlightenment.

The first five stages are connected with moral and mental preparation, and the last three are related to the development of the mind. The development of the mind begins with concentration, which leads to meditation. Meditation gives us enlightenment.

Swami Paramananda said: "The key to concentration is the desire to keep attention on one subject ... When the mind is balanced and well-concentrated, the Higher Self of a person becomes visible ... This means a feeling of oneness with God. The highest form of meditation is to focus on the Absolute Reality, on the Unchangeable."

The philosophy of yoga distinguishes between the mind (Chitta) and the soul (Atman). So, according to Swami Budhananda, "The mind is a subtle body inside a large one. The physical body is just a shell of the mind ... Above the mind, the Atman is the true "I" of man. The body and mind are material, the Atman is pure spirit. The mind is not the Atman, but something else."

Therefore, the highest goal for the Hindu is to purify his spirit and free himself from illusions (Maya) so that the Atman connects with Brahman.

Taoism - the Path to Immortality

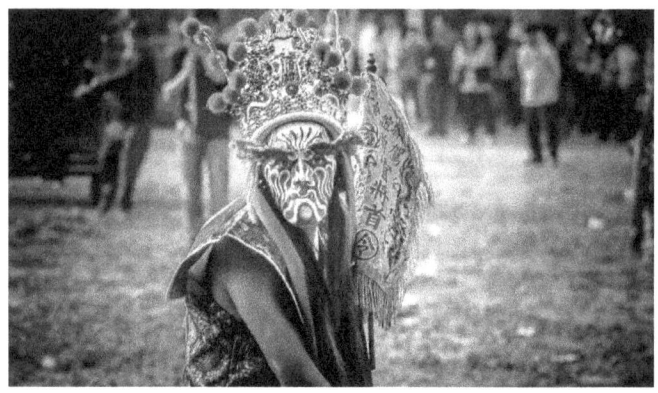

The founder of Taoism is Lao Tzu, who was born in 601 BC. However, many Western scholars studying Chinese texts insist that Taoism as teaching was formed only 300 years after the death of the thinker. At the same time, the followers of Taoism for many centuries believed that this doctrine dates back to the time of the Yellow Emperor Huan Ti, that is, from about the second century.

Despite the fact that no source indicates the mutual influence of Taoism and Hinduism, their philosophical concepts have much in common. While ritualistic Taoism deals with countless gods and goddesses, the philosophical direction teaches the attainment of immortality by merging with Tao.

What is Tao?

Lao Tzu said: "Everything arises from what cannot be called or described because it is beyond the understanding of man; for convenience, it is called Tao." On the Taoist cosmology, the sage said: "Tao creates one. One creates two. Two creates three. Three is the Mother of all things."

The great wisdom contained in these words becomes apparent when we understand that "tao" means the Great Reach, "one" means cosmos, "two" means yin and yang, and "three" means positive, negative and neutral energy charges.

Taoism points the way to the Great Reach, in other words, to gain immortality. How?

Such a question was asked by the Chinese emperor to his teacher Wu Chun Xu, and he answered: "Morality is the first and integral part of the path to immortality. Then the seeker of immortality must meditate on emptiness. Meditating, he combines his mind and breath, eliminates all emotions and worries and focuses his mind on the void. Emptiness is what was before the appearance of being, it is the primordialness of infinity. Return to emptiness means a return to pristine condition."

The Taoist method consists mainly of the development of the "three treasures of man": essence (jing), energy (qi) and mind, or soul (shen).

The Taoist saint of the Ming dynasty, Liu Hua Yang explained: "The secret of developing the pearl of the elixir to achieve holiness is nothing but the function of shen and qi." This means that the secret of immortality lies in meditation aimed at vital energy.

The saint continues the explanation: "The goal of practicing holiness is to transform jing into a sparkling pearl of energy. When this energy passes through different energy points and returns to its energy field, it can be released as an immortal soul. Everyone wants to become a saint, but this method is a mystery of Heaven, so very few have achieved holiness."

Therefore, the highest goal of Taoism is to achieve

immortality, and the main method is meditation, with the help of which the soul returns to emptiness, achieving unity with the Cosmos.

Buddhism - the Path to Nirvana

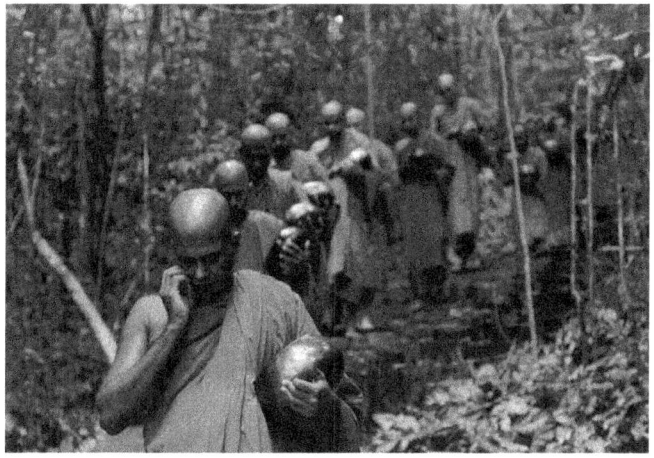

The highest goal of Buddhism is to go to nirvana, that is, to achieve a state where the enlightened mind is freed from the cycle of earthly incarnations. Many great Buddhism teachers have emphasized that meditation is the only path to nirvana. Oddly enough, many Buddhists do not understand the importance of this circumstance. Gautama Buddha himself achieved enlightenment through meditation.

The doctrine and practice of Buddhism resulted in the form of "Ways of eight noble stages." Here they are:

1. correct speech;
2. the right actions;
3. the right way of life;
4. correct views;
5. correct intentions;
6. the correct concentration;
7. the right effort;
8. proper thinking.

The first five stages deal with moral categories and are preparatory for the next three. The last three stages prepare the mind for enlightenment and are realized through meditation. In other words, a Buddhist can do many good deeds, pray to Buddha, become a monk and go to the monastery, but until he meditates, he will not achieve nirvana.

The venerable Dhammananda summarized the purpose of meditation: "First, meditation improves the mind, adapting it to the needs of everyday life, and its highest goal is liberation from the Wheel of Samsara - the cycle of birth and death."

Another great Buddhist teacher said this: "At all times, meditation has been the only means of ultimate comprehension and gaining eternal bliss - the nirvana that the Buddha spoke of."

Zhi Yi, the patriarch of the Chinese Tantai School of Buddhism, said: "Avoid evil deeds, do good, and your soul will find its original, infinite void - this is the teaching of all Buddhas. There are many ways to achieve infinite emptiness, but the main, necessary step is chi-guan.

The same idea was expressed fifteen centuries ago by the venerable Bodhidharma, when the emperor Liang Wu Ti, who became famous for many worthy deeds for the good of the nation, asked him the question: "Sir, considering all the temples that I built, all the Buddhist texts that I translated from Sanskrit, and all the good deeds that I have done in the name of

Buddhism, am I close to nirvana?"

Ji means meditation of rest (samatha), and gu-an means deep meditation (vipassana). These are the two main categories of Buddhist meditation.

The main goal of Buddhism, like Taoism and Hinduism, is to realize the Ultimate Reality, to free oneself from illusions and evil, thus leaving the circle of births and deaths. The path that the great ascetics indicate is the path of meditation.

Christianity - The Kingdom of God

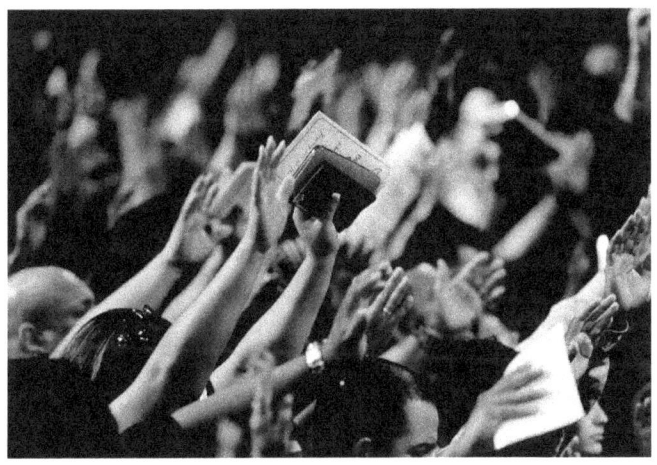

One of the great things about Jesus was the miracles that he did. According to the Bible, Jesus walked on the water, fed five thousand people with five slices of bread and two fish, turned the water into wine and resurrected people. However, the most significant of his miracles were the healings that he performed. He healed for paralysis, lameness, fever, tetanus, hemorrhage, skin diseases, mental disorders, obsession, deafness, and blindness. Many of these healings were done by laying on of hands. We often find mention of this in the New Testament.

Gospel of Luke (chapter 4: 40): "When the sun was

already setting, people brought to Jesus everyone who was sick with various diseases and laying hands on everyone, He healed them."

In the Gospel of Matthew (chap. 8: 14–15), Jesus heals with a touch Peter's mother-in-law from a fever. In the Gospel of Mark (chapters 1: 40–42), Jesus uses hand wrapping to heal a person from leprosy. This is also mentioned in the Gospel of Luke (chapter 5: 2-13). Matthew (chapter 20: 29–34) describes how Jesus healed two blind people by touching their eyes, and in Mark (chapter 8: 22–25), Jesus uses his hands to heal another blind person. In the Gospel of Mark (chap. 7: 32–35), He heals the deaf and dumb with a touch. In the Gospel of Luke (chap. 7: 12–15), Jesus animates a dead person by touching his grave. In Luke (chapter 8: 49–55), Jesus raises a dead girl by touch.

There is so much in common between the laying on of hands that Jesus used and the healing of Reiki. One important similarity is that Jesus could pass on the gift of healing to others. We see in Luke (chapter 9: 1–2) that Jesus gave his twelve apostles the power to cast out all demons and heal diseases. We do not know how

Jesus gave the gift of healing to his apostles, but the very fact of this transmission shows similarities with Reiki.

Another characteristic of Jesus' healing that is similar to Reiki is faith. While faith was required for many of the healings performed by him, it turned out that faith was not required for healing by laying on of hands. Gospel of Mark (chap. 6: 5–6): "He could not have done any other miracle than to lay his hands on several sick people and heal them." And He was struck by the lack of faith in them. So, despite the fact that the sick did not believe, Jesus was still able to heal by laying on of hands. This is one of the important features of Reiki. In order for the treatment to give results, the people receiving it do not need faith.

The fact that Jesus had secret knowledge, which he transmitted only to those to whom he gave the gift of healing, is clearly shown in the Gospel of Matthew (chapter 13: 10–11) and in the gospel of Mark (chapter 4: 10–12, 34). Secret knowledge is also part of Reiki training. For example, this includes symbols and formulas.

It is not known whether Jesus had the gift to heal by touch from birth or acquired it. His life between twelve and thirty years is not described in the New Testament. Some scholars have suggested that Jesus traveled to the East at the time and received secret training in India, Tibet, and China. If so, then it is possible that Jesus went through the initiation of Reiki or something similar, since Reiki originates in these places.

The early followers of the teachings of Jesus formed several groups. One of them was a group of Gnostics. They practiced laying hands and believed that they possessed the secret knowledge that was passed on to them by Jesus and his apostles. Gnostics were divided into smaller groups, some of which are known to us as Docetists, Maronites, and Carpocratians. They were united by deep convictions, which included relying on the personal experience of Jesus, freedom and limited rules, faith in inspiration and inner feelings. Their existence is attested in the Gnostic Gospel, which is part of the Dead Sea Scrolls, as well as in a letter written in the II century by the early father of the Church, Clementius of Alexandria. In his letter, Clementius spoke of the secret Gospel of Mark, which was based on the usual canonical.

In the second century, Christian teaching was centered more on the faith and official doctrines of the Church than on healing or other good deeds and the "inner guidance" used by the Gnostics. At this time, those community leaders who expanded the influence of the church began to subjugate and exterminate those Gnostics who did not submit to the authority of the new Church. With the extermination of the Gnostics and the establishment of the Christian Church, the practice of laying hands was lost by Christians.

Jesus was highly skilled in his skill and was able to heal instantly and with exciting results. Obviously, he perfected a huge amount of metaphysical skills and used them in conjunction to achieve such results.

Was Reiki among those skills? Was Jesus a very high-level Reiki master in addition to being a spiritual teacher?

This cannot be ascertained with absolute accuracy, but the available evidence clearly points to so many similarities that the hands-on healing that Jesus used must have been very closely related to the early form of Reiki. The teachings of Jesus, as well as the examples he demonstrated, are very inspiring. As we continue to improve our spiritual consciousness and allow our inner wisdom to guide us, it is likely that the results will be achieved and, ultimately, we may reach the level that Jesus possessed.

We must remember that the great master of spirituality Jesus said: "Verily I say unto you, anyone who believes in me can perform the same miracles that I did, and even greater ones."

The main goal of Christianity is to return to the Kingdom of God. Despite the fact that in the canonical Christian texts' meditation is not mentioned as a means of spiritual growth, high-level religious practice undoubtedly uses elements of this technique. The following quotes from two prominent Christian saints support this statement.

St. Francis Xavier: "Once after a prayer, I felt filled with bright light, it seemed to me that a veil was falling from my eyes, and before my spiritual gaze all the knowledge accumulated by humanity appeared. Truths that I had no idea about before became obvious and understandable. The state of intuitive perception lasted for twenty-four hours, and when the vision disappeared, I felt my ignorance. At that moment I heard a voice: "Such is mortal human knowledge. Only My Love is worthy of people's attention."

Saint Ignatius: "The mind was suddenly filled with a new and strange light, instantly and for no apparent reason, the secrets of faith and the truth of the universe were revealed to it." The knowledge appeared in such a volume and so distinctly that he thought: "If we put together the spiritual light received by the soul from God over sixty years of life, then all this knowledge could not be compared with what came to me at the time of illumination."

How closely described sensations resemble the experiences of Buddhists, Taoists, Hindus and other mystics! All ecstatic spiritual experiences occurred when the saints were in a state of meditation.

Dr. Johnson, a theologian and Christian bishop who was canonized, writes: "All religions throughout all ages have had their own methods of silent meditation, inner contemplation and the development of spiritual experience ... Representatives of all world religions drew inspiration from internal, spiritual sources. This is confirmed by the historical experience of Christianity and other religious movements.

Obviously, the external form of meditation is not fundamental. It is important that the believer's mind be calm and in contact with God. Sincere prayer is a form of deep meditation."

St. Augustine described the technique and philosophy of Christian meditation. His description erases the line between the Christian and Eastern approaches to reaching the mystical level of perception and gaining an alliance with the Higher Reality. Augustine for a long time preparing himself for spiritual achievement and took the path of self-sacrifice, taming of passions and gaining virtue. Only asceticism and self-discipline can change the character and raise a person to the necessary level of spirituality. Augustine believed that religious contemplation is available only to those who are "cleansed and healed." Contemplation in itself implies "inner self-contemplation" and "prayer concentration." The latter should be accompanied by a concentration of mind and a departure from sensory perceptions. Upon reaching this state, the worshiper must look into his own soul and find a place for God in its depths.

The highest goal of Christian meditation, like Christianity itself, is to enter the Kingdom of God and gain eternal life.

The Gospel of Luke (chapter 17: 20–21) says: "He was asked by the Pharisees when the Kingdom of God came, he answered them: The Kingdom of God will not come in a noticeable way, and they won't say: here it is, or: there. For behold, the kingdom of God is within you."

Islam - Return to God

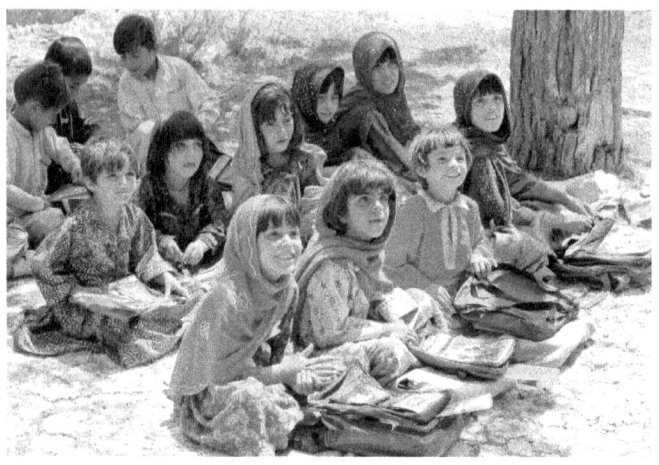

Muslims believe that they live by the breath of Allah. The ultimate goal of Islam is a return to God.

The Islamic religious leader Sheikh Hakim Moinuddin Chishti describes the purpose of Muslims as follows: "Every scripture and every prophet initially says the same thing: we are created by a wise and loving Creator, and the main goal of our existence is to try to find a way to Him. The purpose of our life is to find union with God. "

What are the methods of Islam used to achieve this? Dr. Mir Valiuddin, another prominent Muslim thinker, said that after cleansing the soul and body, "sir" should be freed, that is, combine the mortal with the divine. This is achieved with the help of muraqaba, or contemplation when the soul of a believer is illuminated.

"Muraqaba" means a feeling of Allah's vigilant attention to human affairs. Religious contemplation itself is carried out on two levels, internal and external. External contemplation means "the aversion of the five (organs) of feelings from all that is earthly and the non-manifestation of futile and meaningless emotions in people and in solitude ...".

Inner contemplation means "protecting the soul (heart) from external influences and worthless thoughts about the past or future. During this state, not only vain thoughts but also prayers should be avoided, since everything worldly lowers the level of contemplation." Adherents of Sufism give special attention to meditation.

The Islamic concept of comprehension of God also has much in common with representations of other religious movements.

"Illumination of the spirit" means the overflow of the soul with a sense of Divine Love. Depending on personal qualities, each person is involved in the Universal Spirit. After the spirit has descended upon the body, all worldly relationships and attachments that interfere with its unity with the Supreme should be rejected. Avoid passions and attachments, for they enslave the spirit.

"The One who understands the Truth knows that God is the only existing reality, and everything that is outside of Him is illusory ... The feeling of love manifests itself most fully in the absolute contemplation of the Beloved when the subject does not notice and feels nothing but the object and merges with it completely. This state can be called the apotheosis of Love." Mansur Al-Hallaj expressed this feeling in the following words: "I am the One whom I love, and the One whom I love is Me."

Reiki and Religion

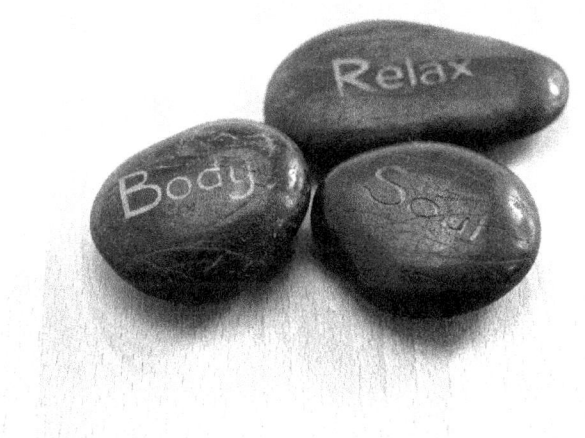

Interestingly, the Reiki art is not tied to any religion. Also, it does not depend on the worldview and the one who sends Reiki energy, and the one who receives it. In this sense, we can say that Reiki art is universal and is available by all, and to all.

REIKI

6 THE FUTURE OF REIKI

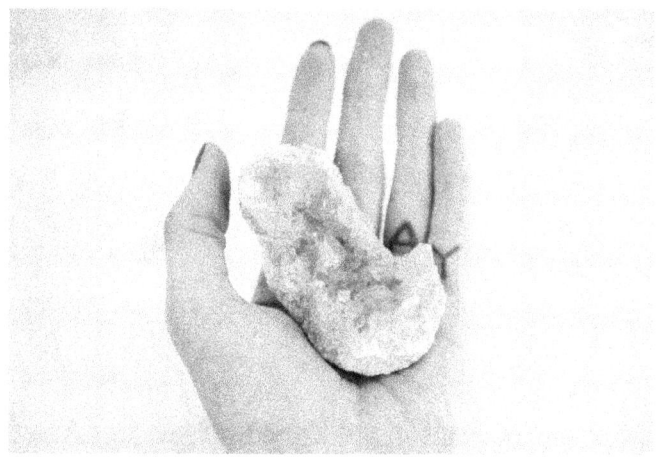

As shown, from time immemorial and to date Reiki is shown to be:

❖ A powerful natural system that opens the flow

of energy through the healer and client;

- ❖ The process of evolution, which increases the natural flow of events, as well as enhances the course of life and affects the achievement of desired goals;

- ❖ A natural healing system that works in perfect harmony with other types of healing;

- ❖ Energy support system, operating with all healing practices;

- ❖ Support for drug treatment that does not conflict with the correct treatment methods. It helps to heal, using the highest internal reserves of the body;

- ❖ Universal healing energy, useful for all forms of life: people, plants, animals and other living things;

- ❖ A permanent way that relieves stress and avoids stressful situations;

- ❖ A well-organized system that perfectly protects against an incorrect reaction to stressful situations;

❖ An effective way to reduce health costs, a way to prevent disease.

However, sometimes it happens that people need to get sick because the disease is also a necessary teacher. It all depends on the spiritual path of a person. Sometimes a person needs to face a disease that will teach him something new, make him understand something.

When you feel good, in good health, you continue to work and do not appeal to your spiritual part. You begin to turn to your spiritual side only when you become ill. Roughly speaking, to take a step forward, you need a good kick in the back. Maybe you need a disease so that you realize something, think about whether you are doing everything right in life. Disease is not such a bad thing. On the contrary, they are a spiritual teacher. Therefore, do not think that getting sick is bad, sometimes even good.

We live in a time of accelerating change, an ever-increasing period of personal and planetary pain. Time began to flow faster due to the displacement of the magnetic poles of the planet, which brought chaos to all levels of life. Disintegration is taking place in countries, people have become hostages in the hands of governments, the number of homeless people is increasing, and the political situation is unstable. The earth is also experiencing a physical crisis, manifested in hurricanes, earthquakes, droughts, fires, volcanic eruptions, destructive tornadoes, floods and landslides that threaten life on the planet. New incurable diseases have appeared, and old diseases and their relapses are becoming increasingly difficult to treat. Our water system is unreliable, and land, water, and air are polluted. Murders, rape, abuse of children become an inevitable part of life.

The old gives way to the new. This is a normal process of rebirth. But the birth of the new must often be accompanied by the dying of the old. We are in the process of dying and are entering the time when the birth of a new life should take place. State leaders and official medicine are not able to alleviate the pain of the planet and people. We all suffer. No one is an exception.

Hate speech, homophobia, religious intolerance, racism - all these are reactions to the pain we experience. So, we are trying to blame someone. All creatures that are now being born are extremely vulnerable, and the possibility of their survival is in question.

But the new is certainly born. There is a growing awareness of the need to cleanse the Earth, the need for change. And although the governments of various countries are completely powerless, and big businesses impede change, they still happen. Political systems die and are reborn in other forms. Beating women, rape, child abuse, incest will soon be a thing of the past. During a crisis, people come together and help each other. They cannot wait for the bureaucrats to finally take action. Governments are forced to take care of their citizens, and not engage in wars.

A new awareness slowly makes its way to the light. Power ceases to be "something outside".

This is best seen in the role women begin to play in modern society. We live in those times when power leaves the hands of a few and becomes the property of all. Increasingly, women are ambiguous in favor of change. They say no to violence and cruelty, they say yes to compassion and peaceful change. Women protest that their bodies, their children and their Earth will be victims of violence. They fight for equality, common sense and universal healing.

There is also the creation of favorable conditions for development. The New Age metaphysical movement provides awareness and promotes the spiritual development of many people. This can trigger the global growth of Human Potential and develop new forms of traditional religions such as Wicca, spiritualism and modern Buddhism. This is a return to the old way of perceiving and thinking, restoring values buried under the rubble of modern life. We will become who we are in reality — mediums, healers, and people who can participate in the conscious Existence.

Many today prefer the ancient methods of healing to modern mechanized medicine. Computerized technology scares away an increasing number of patients with its soullessness and lifelessness. The high prices for medical services, the insurance system and the control of big business and pharmacology tyrants make modern medical methods inaccessible to many people. Standard medicine is not able to answer most questions about the causes of the disease. Now there is a resurgence of therapies taken from the 13th to 17th century by the Inquisition and non-invasive treatments practiced in the past around the world. Herbal medicine, acupuncture, homeopathy, massage - these are just some of them, revived in our days. These methods often help people.

Reiki is one of these methods, perhaps one of the most significant. It does not require any tools and auxiliary means - only the hands of the healer, moreover, Reiki can be used as an addition to other healing systems. This method can be learned easily and quickly - even a child is able to master it. Being simple and deep, the Reiki system teaches us how to heal a disease on a physical, emotional, mental and spiritual level. This is a way of gaining strength in an age of powerlessness and hopelessness. Reiki is a return to the ancient past and the birth of an unknown future.

Reiki teachings emerged from a culture where compassion and unity were valued above all else. Reiki returns the highest values to the Earth. This method is non-invasive and gentle, it will never cause harm or cause pain. In a world full of suffering, Reiki is a refuge for anyone who seeks prosperity. Reiki calms and comforts, relieves pain, stops the blood and brings relief from emotional injuries. Reiki cannot be used for evil, distort or take away from the healer. This method was created for protection, and Reiki Guides know in which world it should be used. The development of Reiki in the West, though, is only in its infancy.

In times of change and violence, Reiki is part of planetary healing. Reiki belongs to everyone and the Earth itself. This is the greatest potential of good that can be given to all the people of the planet. At the dawn of terrestrial cultures, Reiki was a universal system, it was part of our gene code and was woven into DNA molecules. It should not have been lost. The more people who know the Reiki system, the easier the period of earth changes will pass, the less pain and suffering there will be, the easier the birth of a new one will occur. The time has come to bring Reiki to Earth.

This is a call to action addressed to you, women, and to you, understanding men. Time to act for healers and peacemakers - return Reiki to the Earth, as it should have been done a long time ago, begin to heal people, animals and the Earth itself. Let Reiki manifest peace, healing, prosperity and positive change. I urge all Reiki Masters to use their knowledge to its full potential. I ask the Reiki III initiates to relay their skills. And I ask you to learn faster and with an open mindset so that Reiki is available to everyone.

There can be no more excuses and no deferrals. Every day brings ever greater suffering and ever greater pain. The global crisis is getting worse. Remember, kindness, compassion, unity are at the core of Reiki, like all healing. Recognize the need to heal all people during planetary change.

The time has come to heal the Earth, as well as all people and animals.

The time has come.

7 REIKI PRACTICE

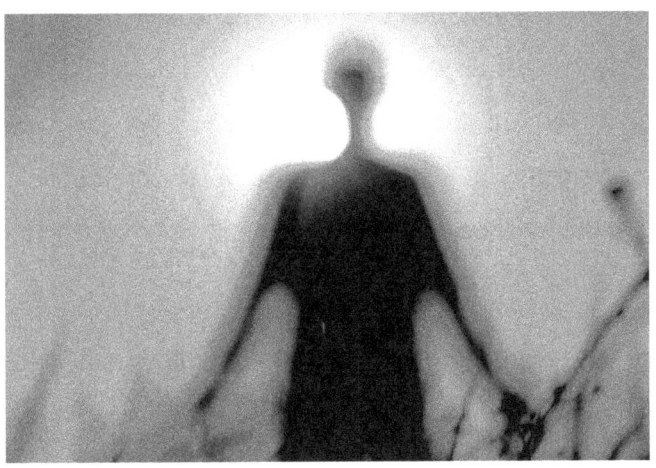

For a full Reiki healing session, you will need a lot of time - an hour or even a little more. To avoid any inconvenience, you need to prepare in advance for this, for which you need to choose the most convenient venue for the session.

It should be noted that if you are conducting a self-healing session, then this is not so important. Such sessions can be carried out while lying in bed - before or after waking up, and even sitting in a comfortable chair while watching TV (of course, you should not watch a football match or a crime chronicle).

But when conducting Reiki healing for another person, a prerequisite is the maximum comfort of both the patient and the healer himself. For almost the entire duration of the session, the patient first lies on his back, and then on his stomach. This may not be very convenient, since it is necessary to observe immobility, and the body becomes numb during a prolonged static state.

It is recommended to place a small pillow under the head of the person being healed so that the neck does not bend much - this position contributes to a better passage of energies through the cervical spine, and the patient does not experience inconvenience during the session. Under slightly bent knees, it is better to place a low roller or a rather tightly rolled blanket. In this position, energy flows freely through the knees and flows freely to the center of the earth through the soles of the feet.

Each specialist selects a massage table for himself since the "right" table greatly facilitates his work. Fatigue of the healer during the session or the uncomfortable position of the patient can nullify all efforts and even cause harm to both the first and second.

During a Reiki healing session, the healer spends a lot of time motionless in each position, and sometimes in several positions, moving only with his hands before moving to another place. Therefore, it will be much more convenient for him to conduct a full session, sitting on a low pillow.

Also, the healer needs to be able to relax his body and find the most comfortable position so as not to interrupt the session due to a cramped arm or a stiff back. This skill is especially important when healing is not carried out on the massage table, but on the bed or on the floor.

Clothing for both the healer and the healed, preferably free cut, comfortable and not restricting movements, made from natural materials. Before the session, the patient should remove the glasses, if they have a pair. Contact lenses can be left, they do not interfere with work.

Sometimes situations arise when it is not possible to conduct a full Reiki session. Then no special preparations are required, the healer acts in a way that will be more convenient and appropriate in each case. For example, returning home after a busy day, you can conduct a healing session to relieve fatigue and recharge energy directly in public transport, without attracting the attention of others. The healer's hands are lying on the navel at this time (in this situation, the person is the healer himself). In general, there are no hard and clear canons for conducting a Reiki healing session. Feel yourself, your sensations, Reiki energy, listen to them and be healed!

With the help of Reiki, you can strengthen your health, both physical and mental, in a fairly short time, change your life for the better, help another person at any time and at any distance. And also, you will find peace, self-confidence and the joy of life.

General Session Rules

1. Entering Reiki Stream

In general, the concept of "entering the Reiki stream" should be taken with a very high degree of conventionality, since there is no literal entry into the word. A person who has been practicing this method of healing for a long time is actually in the Reiki stream constantly, Reiki always surrounds him, every second. And the true meaning of the phrase "enter the Reiki stream" is that the healer is aware of this energy, focuses his attention on the stream and is able to direct it.

In order to enter the stream, it is not necessary to fall into a state of trance, to read Reiki prayers or mantras. Just the healer's clear intention: "I enter the

Reiki stream", "I am in the Reiki stream" or another similar phrase. These words can be pronounced to oneself, can be spoken aloud. It is also allowed to simply feel yourself in a stream of pure energy or imagine yourself standing in it.

Many healers, when entering the energy flow, hold their palms at chest level (Gassho's gesture). There are no clear-cut strict rules and restrictions; everyone chooses a method of entering the Reiki energy flow on their own, guided by their own feelings. The main condition is one: to clearly realize this moment, to formulate a firm intention to enter the stream.

2. Opening the Patient's Aura

This is also nothing super complicated. The healer makes a hand movement over the patient, similar to the way the curtain is opened. "Opening the curtain" is allowed with either hand. And in this case, as when entering the stream, the main work consists precisely in the intent of the healer. He makes a movement of his hand in order to help himself to form his intention more clearly.

However, if for some reason he did not make such a movement, then there is nothing wrong with that. The patient's aura will open itself, without any physical efforts on the part of the healer, only his intent is enough.

3. Passing Reiki Flow Through a Patient

In preparation for the session, it is necessary to let the Reiki energy flow through the patient whole, from top to bottom.

If a person is in a prone position, the healer runs his hands along his body from top to bottom, at a distance of 30–35 cm several times (the number is arbitrary). If the patient is sitting, you need to put your hands on his shoulders and let the Reiki flow through him. At this stage, the healer, as a rule, simultaneously conducts a general diagnosis of the patient. There are no age restrictions for Reiki classes, you can attend them from birth. Moreover, there are special programs for pregnant and very young children, aimed at their development and health. But initiation to Reiki is strongly discouraged until 7 years old until the time for self-awareness begins.

4. Forming Intentions When Conducting a Session with a Patient

Reiki energy is universal, it contains information about all phenomena, in particular, about how a human body should be in a state of complete health. Some time ago it was believed that Reiki energy constantly surrounds a person, he is in this stream always and everywhere. However, until the healer has formed an intention, the energy flow of Reiki is dissipated. And it is his intention that allows you to focus Reiki, direct the flow to those problematic places in the body that need to be healed.

Of course, it is possible to conduct a general healing session for the patient, passing, in turn, all the positions of the laying on of hands. In this case, the energy of Reiki will correct what is not in order in the body. But if a person has a specific problem (for example, chronic headache, diseases of other organs), then it is desirable, and even necessary, to work it out purposefully, for which the healer forms the intention.

The intention is always neutral and sounds something like this: "I (the healer) direct the energy of Reiki to relieve the spasm of the brain vessels of the (patient), its general healing (of the patient)", etc. Thus, intention is the main goal of the Reiki session.

But when forming an affirmation, it should be firmly remembered that in no case should there be words of negation and bearing a negative meaning.

All of the above, of course, does not mean that during the session the energy will be directed to the solution of a specific voiced problem. Unlike the healer and patient, as already mentioned, Reiki has complete information about the health status of each person. Therefore, during a session, Reiki heals, trying to bring maximum benefit to a person. And if in the process of healing the healer feels that it is necessary to hold his hands longer in any particular place, then this feeling must be heeded.

At this stage of the session, hands are laid on all positions, together with the fifth stage.

When forming any affirmation, remember: simplicity and conciseness of intention bring maximum effect, and vice versa, extended affirmations with a vague goal lose their emotional strength.

5. Forming a Message to End the Session with the Patient

The Reiki message is a kind of affirmation in which the final result of the session is formulated. The healer uses this message to enhance the effect of the session. It is always pronounced in a positive manner in the present tense. This is an image of the end result of a session. During a session, the intent and message of the healer may sound like this.

Intention: "I fill him (her) - the name of the patient - with energy, give him (her) strength."

Message: "He (she) - the name of the patient - is healthy and energetic."

When conducting a self-healing session, affirmations can be as follows.

Intention: "I fill myself with energy, give myself strength."

Message: "I feel great, I am healthy and energetic." After completing all the positions, the healer forms the message again, symbolically closes the patient's aura and ends the session. If in his work the healer uses Reiki symbols (these are healers of the second level and higher), then they are visualized and superimposed on the patient, after forming the intention, immediately before the message.

REIKI

8 THE REIKI HEALING SESSION

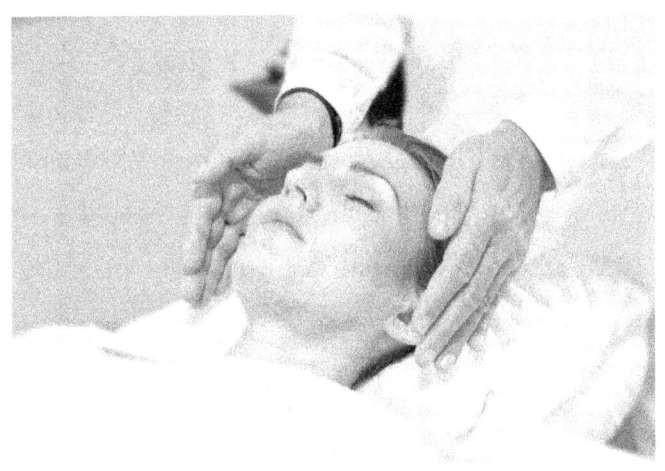

Guide to Physical, Emotional and Mental and Spiritual Healing

Reiki's benefits are enormous. It helps in the healing of diseases in all respects: both physical, and mental, and emotional, and spiritual. It relieves physical and emotional stress, bringing complete relaxation. It cleanses the body of accumulated toxins and helps get rid of bad habits and addictions. Reiki enhances a person's creativity and energy. It improves memory and creates a positive attitude. It also helps a person overcome anger and fear within himself and live in peace and harmony with the people around him. In addition, it helps in the treatment of diseases such as insomnia, overweight, lethargy, fatigue, migraine, and strengthens a person's faith in himself.

When performing hand positions in Reiki, a specific sequence is always used. During a Reiki session, three areas are distinguished: head, front of the body, and rear of the body. In each of them, four to five positions are identified, called the main ones. Healing should be started at these positions from the head, gradually descending to the feet from the front of the body, and then from head to feet from the back.

There is an important condition: the healer should never conduct a session until his hands are warm enough. Cold hands will cause the patient only unpleasant sensations, and in addition, through them the discharge of cold (negative) energy into the patient's body is possible.

In Reiki, the healer always uses both hands, placing them with palms down. The fingers are straightened and tightly closed.

Hands are placed in the desired position gently, relaxed, without pressure. After the healer's hands rest on the patient's body, Reiki's energy begins to flow automatically.

During the session, both the healer and the patient physically sense the passing stream of Reiki energy. But these feelings, as a rule, are always different. If the patient's body needs cold, then he will feel cool. And the healer at the same time may feel that his hands are very hot. It feels like one Reiki session is almost never like another. Each time, these sensations change both in the patient and in the healer. It is impossible to predict them, but they are always present.

In general, it should be emphasized that there are no right and wrong ways to conduct a Reiki session. Always in the first place, it is necessary to be guided by your intuition and feelings. If you suddenly feel that you should skip a certain position, feel free to do it, your body knows better what it needs at the moment. Quite often during the session, there is a feeling that the hands seemed to be glued to one place. Do not try to "unstick" them, keep your hands on this part of the body until this feeling disappears, and only then move on to the next positions.

During the entire session, it is necessary to ensure that when laying on, the arms are not crossed (both during healing and self-healing), since this position of the limbs interferes with the free flow of energy.

Healing should be started from the head, gradually descending to the feet from the front of the body, and then from head to feet from the back.

With the help of Reiki energy, it is possible to heal a person not only physically, but also on a more subtle spiritual level. An experienced healer, located on the upper steps of Reiki, is able to correct bad karma, balance the chakras, and purify the aura. But such effects require much more time compared with the treatment of diseases of the physical body.

Self-Healing

By familiarizing yourself with the general principles and rules of conducting a Reiki session, you can begin the process of self-healing.

Before starting a session, it is advisable to meditate, ask for help and protection. So, always start a self-healing session from the head.

1.) The first position is to straighten the palms of the hands with closed fingers gently over your eyes and hold for 5 minutes, the time can vary slightly depending on the sensations. This position perfectly helps to relieve headaches of a different nature, relieve eye strain. It is used in the treatment of ear, throat, and nose, all kinds of lymphatic diseases, the area of the "third eye".

Performing the first position helps with colds, relaxes the entire body. It also relieves stress, sharpens intuition, and has a beneficial effect on the growth of a person's spirituality. It has an effect directly on the sixth chakra.

2.) The second position - put your hands on both sides of the face, with your palms wrapping around your cheeks, thumbs under your ears, middle and index fingers lying on your temples. The implementation of this position eliminates headache and ear pain, fatigue, relieves stress, helps in solving problems associated with the immune system, nerves. It also improves mental and emotional state, memory. It can be used with the help of the dying. It also affects the sixth chakra.

3.) The third position - move your hands to the back of the head. In this position, you embrace the Crown and Third Eye chakra from behind. Performing this position helps in the treatment of headache, neck, and back, colds, spine, relieves stress.

The energy received at this position normalizes weight, relieves fears, reduces nervous tension, improves your perception of color, speech abilities, and enhances insight. Like the previous two, in the subtle plane, it affects the sixth chakra.

You should work out this position for about 5 minutes.

4.) Fourth position, throat. The position helps to cure diseases of the throat and thyroid gland.

Performing this position, you remove emotional blocks, gain greater self-confidence, and strengthen your creative abilities. On the subtle plane, the throat position affects the fifth chakra.

5.) Fifth position - The next, cordial position is used only for self-healing. It is performed on the chest. Place your palms slightly above your chest, in the heart region. It helps in the treatment of lung diseases, diseases of the cardiovascular system. This position cures of deep grievances, causes a feeling of love, trust, spiritual harmony, gives joy.

6.) Next, follow the position of the solar plexus. To do this, move your arms lower than in the cardiac position, put on the ribs under the chest. This position helps to cure diseases of the liver, gall bladder, stomach, spleen. When fulfilling the position of the solar plexus, the will strengthens, fears disappear, it is possible to get rid of stress, relax, tune in to the energy of the Universe. It affects the third chakra.

7.) The position of the abdomen. Keeping the position of the palms the same as in the position of the solar plexus, lower your hands to the middle of the abdomen, to the navel, one palm lower. This position affects the second chakra. Helps in the treatment of kidneys, adrenal glands, digestive organs, liver. At the mental level - depressive states, emptiness, inability to feel happiness.

Getting energy in this position, you can get rid of constant anxiety, dissatisfaction, become more confident in yourself and calmer.

8.) You can use the eighth position only for self-healing since in this position the hands touch the genital area. In this position, place your hands one above the other just above the pubic bone.

Performing an inguinal position helps to cure diseases of the kidneys, adrenal glands, ovaries in women, helps to eliminate problems in the genitourinary system, relieve emotional and physical fatigue. It also eliminates sexual fears and brings natural sexuality into a state of harmony. Getting the energy of Reiki in this position, you will accelerate the healing of the colon and small intestine, intestines, bladder, genitals. It has a direct effect on a subtle level on the first and second chakras.

After completing the Reiki positions on the head and front of the body, you can move on to the knees, ankles, and feet. (But we consider it necessary to note that these positions do not belong to the positions of traditional Reiki, therefore, they are often missed.)

If you nevertheless decided to hold such positions, you need to accept the sitting position.

First act on your knees. To do this, put your hands on the front of both knees: the left hand lies on the left knee, the right hand on the right. The position can be performed sitting on a chair or lying on its side, or on its back, legs tucked up. Performing this position helps with headaches, knee injuries, stagnation in the neck, energy blockade observed in the lower body.

Next, go to the ankle joints. It is possible to perform a position both simultaneously on both legs, and alternately, sitting or lying at your request. On each joint, the lead time is 5 minutes. You can also combine this position with the previous one by placing your left hand on your left knee and your right hand on your left ankle. After 5 minutes, change legs: put your right hand on your right knee, left - on your right ankle. Perform for 5 minutes. The position assists in the treatment of the thyroid gland, throat, and lymph nodes. It also helps unlock energy.

When finished, go to the foot position. Here, as in some previous positions, two options are acceptable: the first - the left hand grasps the left foot, the right - the right foot. In the second option, the foot of each leg is clasped with both hands. Choose the option that is most convenient for you. At the same time, you can both sit and lie on your back with legs crossed, placing your feet in the middle of your hands. On the feet there are areas associated with all the organs of our body, when exposed to them, a healing effect on the body as a whole will be caused. Also, the fulfillment of this position has an effect on a subtle level on all chakras.

Next, the self-healing session goes to the back of the body. Start completing positions also from the head. The positions for the back are similar to those performed for the front of the body.

First, you hold a position in which you put one hand on the back of the head and the other on the crown (parietal chakra). Or both hands are allowed on the parietal chakra.

If you suddenly fell asleep during a self-healing session, this is not at all scary. The power of Reiki heals no matter what state you are at this moment, energy continues to flow into the organism, positively affecting all problem areas and organs.

9.) The next position is for the back of the neck and upper part of the shoulder girdle. Many people in this area are very stressed and often have pain. Holding this position helps to cope with them, as well as relax and overcome stress. Influence on the subtle plane is on the fifth chakra.

10.) In the next position above the ribs, below the shoulder blades, on the back of the heart chakra, place your palms so that they look at each other.

The action of this position is similar to the action of the position of the solar plexus. It also helps to get out of stress, relieves of various fears, and strengthens willpower. At a subtle level, it affects the third chakra.

11.) Without changing the position of the hands, lower them a little lower on the lower back, and perform a position on the lumbar. It is very effective in diseases of the kidneys and abdominal organs. It affects the second or third chakras.

12.) Then, without changing the position of the hands, move them to the lower back (sacrum). Performing this position helps to cure the intestines, genital area, and tailbone injuries. It also affects the first and second chakras.

At the end of the session, repeat the position for the legs, with the only difference being that put your hands on the back of the legs, including the feet.

Healing Other People

A Reiki session for another person is practically no different from a self-healing session, there are only a few nuances. Each position, as in self-healing, takes about 5 minutes.

The healer's hands during the treatment of the patient are directed outward by the palms, which slightly changes the performance of certain positions. But most importantly, the healer should be extremely discreet and not invade the patient's intimate areas. This condition makes it impossible to use some items.

As already mentioned above, crossing the arms and legs of both the healer and the healed is unacceptable. This position of the limbs prevents the passage of energy and significantly reduces the positive effect of treatment.

A session begins, as in self-healing, from the head. First, the healer gently puts concave palms over the patient's eyes. Then he moves his hands on the cheeks of the patient, easily resting his little fingers on his ears. In the third position, the healer slightly lifts the healed head, putting his hands under it.

When performing the throat position, the healer can place his hands just below the throat, on the collarbone of the healed. This is due to the fact that a fairly large number of people experience discomfort if they feel the hands of an outsider on their throats. In order to perform the next position, the healer must be located on the side of the patient. It should be noted that this position can be skipped if the patient is a woman and she feels uncomfortable.

The next position is the fifth, carried out on the lower ribs under the chest.

Next, the healer performs the position of the abdomen, the sixth position, and then all the same positions as during the self-healing session.

After completing all the positions on the front side of the body, the healer asks the patient to roll over on his stomach and continues the session on the back side. The positions on the head are the same as in self-healing.

The healer holds positions on the upper thoracic spine, the seventh position, descends without changing the position of the hands, on the lower thoracic part, the eighth position, and then on the lumbar, the ninth position.

Then he puts his hands on the popliteal region, tenth position, ankle joints, ankles and feet of the healed, eleventh position.

Sometimes it happens that the healed is so seriously ill that there is no way to turn him on his stomach. In such a situation, the healer performs positions only on one side of the body. Such an option is also possible - to conduct a session with another person not in all positions, but with hands on only the area of pain.

During a Reiki session, the healer does not give up his energy, unlike healing with the help of extrasensory abilities - he allows the channel to appear through which the vital energy will flow to the healed.

Due to various reasons and circumstances, not every person can give his body a full course of Reiki healing. In this situation, you can go through a short session, which takes less time and does not cover all positions. Of course, a full treatment is preferable, but it is better to at least do something for the person's physical health and spiritual development than to remain inactive, referring to all kinds of difficulties.

Short Reiki Healing Session

1. The healer puts his hands on the shoulders of the healed and makes contact with him.

2. Next, he puts his hands on the parietal part of the head, leaving open the seventh, crown chakra.

3. The healer places one hand on the patient's forehead and the other on the neck, in the region of the brain.

4. Next, he moves one hand to the seventh cervical vertebra, the second to the cavity under the Adam's apple.

5. Then, without changing the position of the hands, lower them to the sternum and between the shoulder blades at the same level.

6. The healer puts one hand on the solar plexus, and the other on the back at the same level.

7. The healer places one hand under the navel of the patient, the other on the sacral region.

8. Then he puts one hand on the right knee of the healed, and the other on his sacrum. Then performs the same position on the left knee.

9. At the end of the session, the healer puts his hands on top of the patient's feet.

Group Healing

This is one of the peculiarities of Reiki. It is possible to practice group Reiki treatments in order to harmonize and reinforce the energy of all the people of the group. One of the goals of Reiki exchange groups is to allow beginners to understand Reiki receiving from those already initiated into Reiki. The Reiki exchange will allow the various participants to express their feelings and to discover the important potential of energy transfer during a Reiki sharing.

Many practitioners of Reiki techniques offer Reiki exchange sessions, this is one of the strengths of Reiki, an important community open to sharing and exchange of treatment. Those wishing to discover Reiki thus have the opportunity to meet and interact with people who already have experience (people at levels 1, 2, 3).

The Reiki Masters generally offer their students Reiki exchanges between initiates and practitioners in order to allow the practice of Reiki within a group. These workshops are generally open to everyone.

A Reiki exchange always has a learning purpose. Either it is to learn to lay hands and develop confidence in the practice of caring for others. Either it is through the exchange to receive a particular teaching specific to each. Each participant usually receives care from the whole group in turn. Participants learn the different positions of the hands in a Reiki group exchange. The

Reiki exchange allows you to compare your own techniques with those of other participants. The richness of these exchanges allows each participant to find a pleasant and friendly environment to progress in the technique and in the felt.

Generally, the principle is as follows: "sometimes we are in a physical, emotional or mentally difficult state and support would be welcome. You will receive energy from a group of people and it will help you recover, but it does not mean that you will not be able to engage in your own healing process with concrete and positive thinking, because true healing does not 'happen' and can come only from you." - Eric Micha'el Leventhal.

9 REIKI WITH CRYSTALS

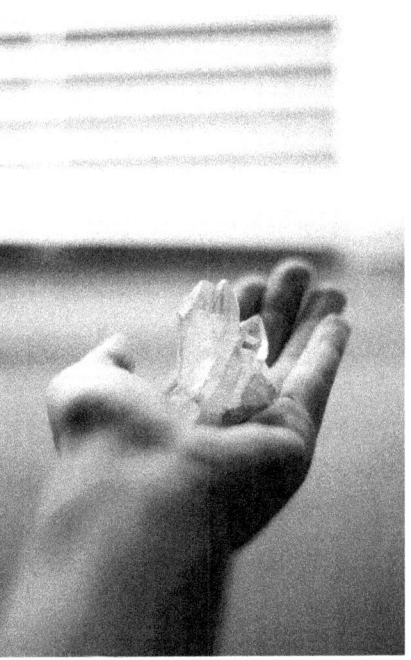

Reiki is combined with many oriental methods of treatment, including treatment with stones, crystals. The crystals contain energy that affects the human body along with the energy of the hands. With the help of Reiki and crystals, it is possible to eliminate the effects of emotional stress, restore physical strength, overcome the strip of failures, and protect yourself from adverse environmental factors.

For centuries, man has been extracting crystals from the earth. In recent years, artificial crystals grown by special technologies have been increasingly used for various purposes. Crystals are composed of molecules of geometric structure. They are ordered in such a way that they form symmetrical shapes.

Crystals are able to grow and accumulate information in themselves. Their energy matrix is used to treat many diseases. The energy of crystals penetrates through the subtle bodies into the physical body, and also acts on the mental level. To the greatest extent, crystals act on bodies, they concentrate energy in blocked zones and then contribute to its dispersion. Thus, crystals eliminate blocks in the body's energy system. They help strengthen a person's own energy and use it more efficiently, for the benefit of their own personality. However, they do not change the characteristics of thinking, do not prevent the appearance of negative thoughts, and after them the corresponding emotions. In this case, Reiki harmoniously complements the effect of crystallotherapy.

Crystals are used in combination with Reiki in many ways. In practice, Reiki of the first stage, the crystals are charged with energy, holding them in their hands. These crystals can be used personally or transferred to a sick person who will wear them on the body, used for meditation. In practice, second-level Reiki, crystals are charged in various ways and treated at a distance. For this, not only the energy transmitted by the hand is used, but also directed thoughts. The most complete effect of the treatment with stones and crystals is achieved in a state of meditation.

Crystals and stones are also feedback. With prolonged wear on the body, they can change color, become smoother or rougher. This indicates a change in energy status and health. Of great importance for the treatment is the choice of a suitable crystal that can resonate with the patient's energy field. Sometimes, in choosing a crystal, rely on intuition, which the Reiki master has well developed.

For treatment, crystals are often selected depending on the disease and place of application, and their color also matters. Color perception tunes the body in a certain way, especially it affects the psycho-emotional sphere. Often crystals are selected according to the color in accordance with the color of the chakras.

For the first chakra (muladhara), red and black crystals are used (black tourmaline, rhodonite, pomegranate, bloody jasper, hematite).

Crystals of orange and brown color (tiger eye, aventurine, carnelian) are suitable for the second chakra (svadhisthana).

The third chakra (manipura) is healed with yellow stones (aventurine, citrine, amber).

The fourth chakra (anahata) is combined with

amazonite, rose quartz, malachite.

For the fifth chakra (vishudha) use stones of blue color (amazonite, turquoise).

In the area of the sixth chakra (ajna), amethyst, lapis lazuli, fluorite are applied.

The seventh chakra (sahasrara) is exposed to the positive effects of amethyst, rock crystal.

There are universal crystals that are effective for all chakras. These include rock crystal, rose quartz, amethyst, citrine, rauchtopaz. You can use both polished, faceted stones and crystals, as well as in its natural form.

After unfolding the crystals on the patient's body, the Reiki master charges stones by alternately applying his palms. After each session, they are cleaned.

Red Stones

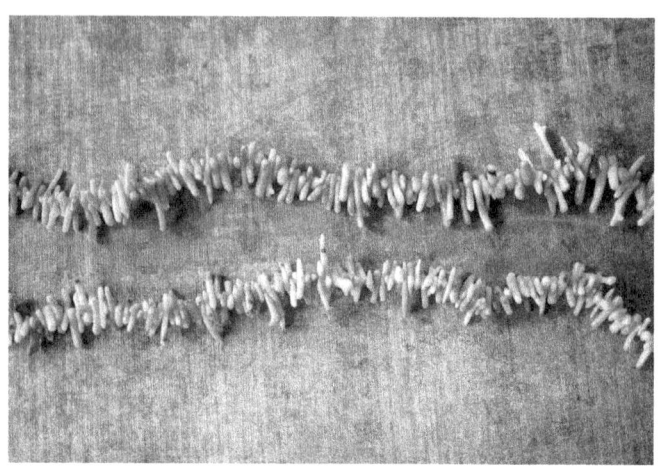

Ruby, pomegranate (almandine, pyrope), red rhodonites, tourmalines, agates, carnelian (carneols), opals, zircons, rhodochrosites, jasper, amber, corals, obsidian.

The red color is traditionally in many cultures a symbol of fire, blood, life, the universe itself. It also represents the color of an active life position, energy and power.

Features of red color made it one of the most popular in folk medicine. It has primarily an exciting and irritating effect. The red color has a particularly powerful effect on the process of hematopoiesis, stimulating an increase in the number of red blood cells, blood cells and increasing the level of hemoglobin in the blood. Modern studies have shown that red color is extremely beneficial for red bone marrow - one of the main organs of blood formation.

Even the ancient healers of the East noticed the effectiveness of red stones in the fight against infectious viral diseases. They are recommended for improving vision, eliminating headaches, as well as certain skin diseases (e.g. measles, chickenpox, etc.). In the Middle Ages, red stones were used to treat scarlet fever. They help a lot in relieving headaches. In medical cosmetology, red crystals are often used to improve skin color.

The impact of red stones is extremely diverse. In addition to the above areas, they are used in folk and official stone therapy (treatment with stones) for neuropsychiatric diseases. Their effectiveness has long been proven in the event of a breakdown, apathy, and depressive states. Red stones can cause a person to feel confident in their abilities and safety, create an optimistic mood. They stimulate the work of the brain well, relieve lethargy and drowsiness, activate sexuality, thus helping to solve many problems associated with the reproductive system, even such as infertility.

Pink Stones

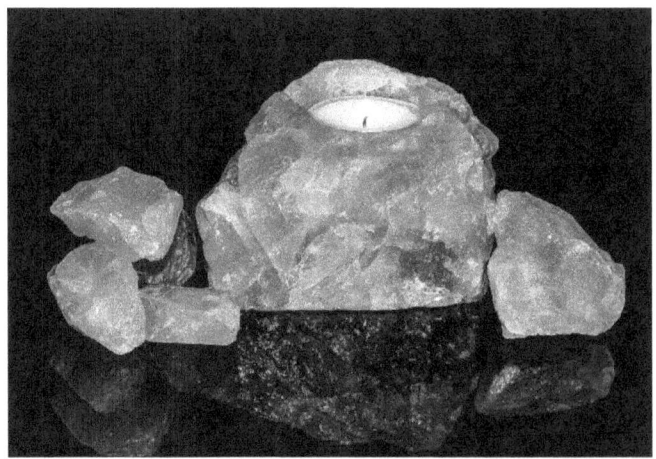

Garnet (rhodolite), morganite (sparrow), pink topazes, sapphires, tourmalines (rubellites), quartz, coral, rhodonites, rhodochrosites, fluorites, sodalites, spinel, pearls.

Pink color is the color of love, tenderness, sensuality. Compared to red, it has a much milder effect on the human body. It calms and relaxes well both physically and psychologically. Therefore, all shades of pink are widely used in Reiki and psychotherapy. Pink stones are often used to normalize the activity of the endocrine system and endocrine glands.

Studies have shown that regular wearing or contemplation of pink gems strengthens the immune system, improves the quality of vision and hearing. Especially often in medical practice, rose quartz is used. In ancient times, it was often called the heart stone.

Orange Stones

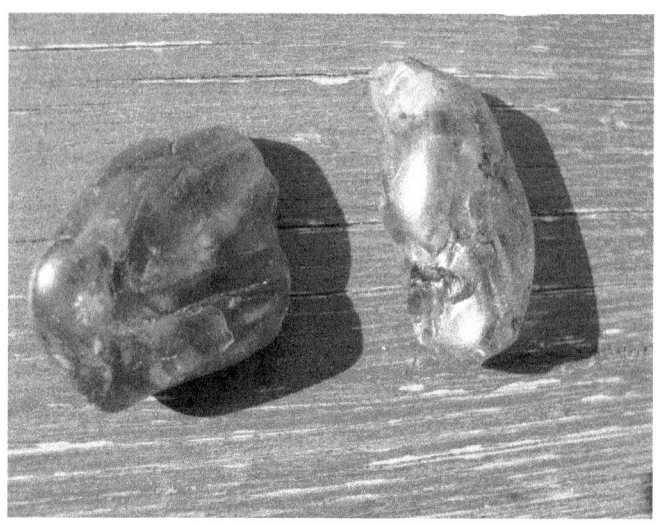

Hyacinth (citrine orange), orange agates, carnelian, sardonyxes, opals, pomegranates (Hessonites), amber, jasper, heliolite (sun stone), Altai quartzites.

In ancient times, the orange color was most often personified with the living Sun, which gave life to all. Like red, it is the color of energy and is capable of exerting a very powerful effect on the human body.

Accordingly, this color gives health, vitality, energy, youth, and beauty. Orange stones have long been used to treat a wide variety of diseases.

One of the most common ailments that were treated with their help back in the Middle Ages includes diseases related to the genitourinary sphere. The warm orange color of crystals and minerals has a generally warming effect. At the same time, it serves as a powerful source of energy for the genitals, stimulating sexuality in women and increasing potency in men.

Orange color also contributes to the regeneration and rejuvenation of various body tissues. It has a beneficial effect on the circulatory system and the condition of the skin.

Extremely useful orange color in the treatment of almost all organs of the respiratory system of the body: larynx, pharynx, trachea, bronchi, lungs. Orange stones help to cure not only inflammation of the throat, tonsillitis, bronchitis, etc., but they can also significantly help even people suffering from bronchial asthma.

Orange color activates and regulates many metabolic

processes in the body, including the action of the endocrine glands. The healing effects of orange amber, jasper, agates, carnelian, hessonites (yellow pomegranates) on the state of the endocrine glands have long been proven.

In Ayurvedic medicine of the East, a special place is occupied by orange-red opals, which are attributed to the stones of God and love. It is believed that they are extremely useful in chronic diseases that are accompanied by large accumulations of mucus in the body.

Orange stones are a wonderful tool in the fight against depression, chronic fatigue syndrome, melancholy. Regular contemplation of amber, jasper, citrines, and other "sun" stones promotes the production of pleasure hormones - endorphins, which not only increase mood but also strengthen the body's protective functions. They are also indispensable for maintaining and increasing overall tone.

Yellow Stones

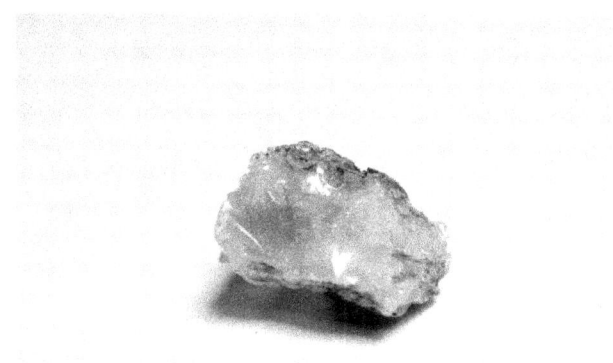

Beryl, chrysoberyl, golden yellow tiger eye, yellow sapphires, topazes, tourmalines (dravites), agates, hyacinths, citrines, heliodors, opals, jades, spinel, fluorites, zircons, carnelian, jasper, amber.

Since ancient times, yellow has been considered the color of the sun and life. The sun is the source of life on Earth. Thanks to it, herbs and trees grow and bear fruit, it gives warmth to animals and people.

This color is extremely important for the life of the human body. Yellow is a wonderful natural tonic. It activates the central nervous system, positively affects the brain, improving mental potential. Yellow stones are especially useful as a remedy for psychophysiological overwork, nervous and physical exhaustion, as well as apathy, depression, stress, and other negative environmental influences. Yellow crystals help relieve tension, depression, increase mood, self-confidence and inner self-esteem of a person.

The constant wearing of yellow stones improves the quality of memory and allows you to speed up the process of assimilation of new information.

All shades of yellow have an amazing property: they simultaneously contribute to concentration and concentration of attention and increase activity, help solve problems with overweight.

The contemplation of yellow gems improves vision. They are used in the treatment of eye diseases associated with impaired vascular function, damage to the retina, strabismus, etc.

Amber has been especially popular among yellow

stones for several millennia. Petrified resin for many, many centuries, pine resin contains a unique natural bio stimulant - succinic acid, which can have a beneficial effect on many internal processes that occur in the body.

The scope of amber in medicine is extremely diverse. It is used in the treatment of diseases of internal organs (especially the liver, kidneys, thyroid gland, throat), joints, skin. Petrified resin has a positive effect on infectious and viral diseases.

Yellow stones are very popular in the treatment of nervous and mental illnesses, as they can have a calming and balancing effect.

Green Stones

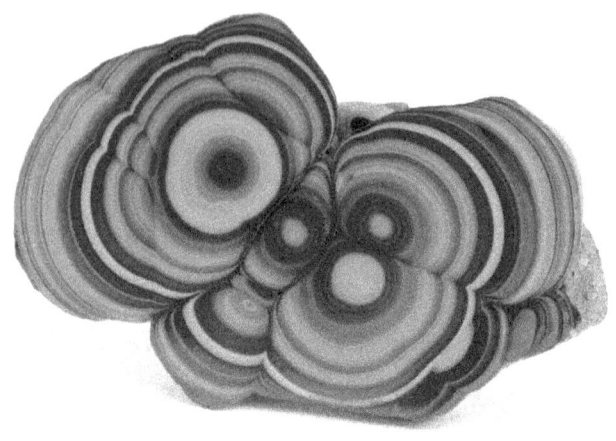

Emeralds, chrysoprase, turquoise, amazonite, serpentine, jadeite, malachite, cat's eye, aventurines, alexandrites, green garnets (andradite, uvarovit, demantoid, etc.), aquamarines, nephrites, tourmalines, fluorites, chrysolites, chrysolites, spinel, jasper.

Green is the color of the rebirth of life and the universe, peace, and happiness. This is one of the most common and important colors of wildlife. It also personifies the color of harmony both within a person and in his relations with the outside world.

Green color has a wide range of healing effects. It maintains an optimal physical and psychological state, has a calming effect and at the same time prevents fatigue and increases vitality and performance.

Thanks to the refreshing, calming and pacifying effect, traditional healers of the East and West have long used the green color to treat increased emotional arousal, imbalance, and temper, various nervous and mental disorders of both adults and children.

The quality of an emerald is determined by its color, not its transparency. Dark green emeralds are valued even above the diamond. The authenticity of the stone is confirmed by splits, the smallest cracks, defects, and foreign inclusions. Their absence suggests that the crystal is not of natural origin, but a skillful fake.

Green stones are currently widely used in stone therapy. They extremely beneficially affect excitable, nervous children, pregnant women, people suffering from various phobias. These are some of the most powerful antidepressants that help create a cheerful mood and increase self-confidence.

The effectiveness of using green minerals as an anesthetic has long been known. Green turquoise in the East has often been used as part of medicines prepared to treat eye diseases.

In the Middle Ages, green olivine in the countries of the Mediterranean and Western Asia was considered one of the most effective means to strengthen male potency.

Aquamarine also has a beneficial effect on the functioning of the brain. In medieval medicine of the East, diamonds with a greenish tint were recommended for use during a difficult pregnancy and as a means of facilitating the process of childbirth.

One of the most powerful in terms of energy and, accordingly, healing effects on the human body has long been considered a serpentine - a stone of dark green color with a specific pattern resembling snake skin. It is widely used to treat both physical and mental ailments. It is effective as a firming and tonic for debilitated and debilitated patients.

Serpentine in antiquity and the Middle Ages among many peoples of the East and West was considered one of the most powerful antidotes that could draw poison from wounds received from snake bites, scorpions and various poisonous insects. Healers also recommended its constant wearing to people suffering from frequent headaches.

Green stones are widely used to get rid of ailments of the musculoskeletal system, especially the spine, as well as for fractures of the extremities to accelerate the process of regeneration and restoration of broken bones and mobility of the limbs.

They also help with disorders of the gastrointestinal tract (including constipation and diarrhea), impaired liver function. Doctors of the East used them for diseases of the gallbladder and spleen.

It is extremely beneficial for the eyes to regularly contemplate stones of green color, as they relieve muscle tension and overwork, thereby contributing to better vision. The famous Arab philosopher and physician Abu Reyhan Biruni, for example, believed that regular contemplation of beryl strengthens vision.

Some green stones, for example, heliotrope (green jasper with red splashes), have a blood-purifying and hemostatic effect. Therefore, it is often used for anemia. The ancient healers of Europe and Asia often used alexandrite to strengthen the heart, blood vessels and improve the process of hematopoiesis.

Jade, tourmaline, malachite, serpentines are able to heal open wounds and long healing ulcers. They are useful in some skin diseases (for example, eczema).

Many green stones are used to remove poisons and toxins from the body. Due to their properties, they retain youth, freshness, and beauty (especially skin and hair) longer, they have also been widely used in cosmetology.

Blue and Cyan Stones

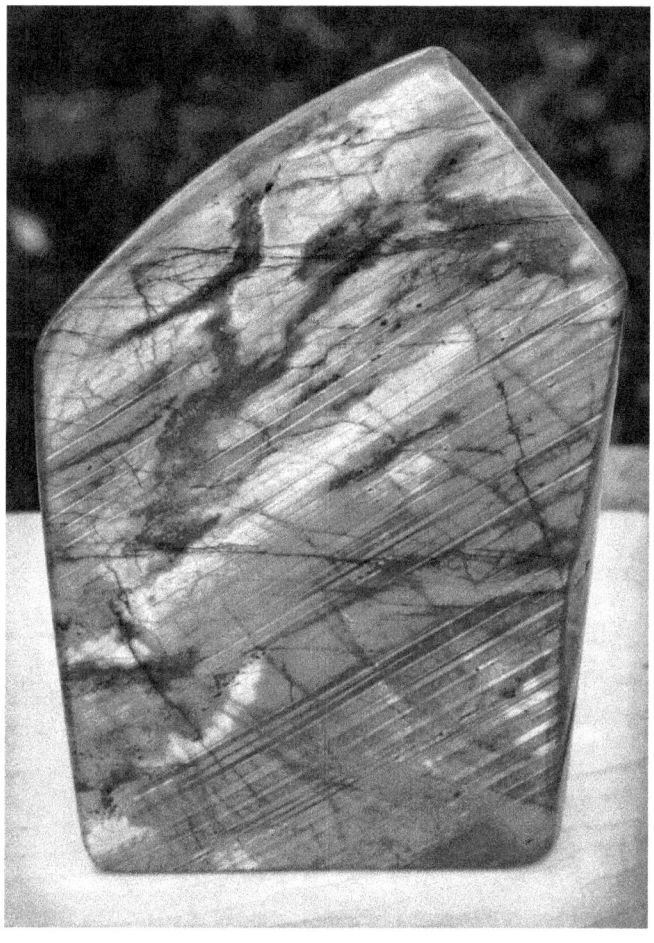

Lapis lazuli, turquoise, aquamarines, amazonites, blue sapphires, topazes, tourmalines, azurites, iolites, blue opals, zircons, fluorites, chalcedony (sapphirins), agates, spinel, hawkeye, labradorites, sodalites.

Blue and cyan have always been associated with the color of air, water, ice, cold. They personify spirituality, romance, contemplation, clarity, and perfection.

For several millennia, blue and cyan have been recognized as healers in folk medicine. The scope of their application is extremely vast. Blue and cyan tones have a calming effect on the human body, relieve physical and psychological fatigue, have a powerful antidepressant effect, help with insomnia, increased emotional and mental excitability, in overcoming various fears, relieving strong nervous attacks, aggressive and anxiety states, etc. The psychotherapeutic effect of blue and blue crystals and minerals has been used for many centuries in meditation, to enhance creativity and intuition.

In psychotherapy, they have been used for a long time with hypochondria, melancholy, hysterical conditions, dementia (including senile). From time immemorial, traditional healers have used dark blue and especially blue-green stones for the treatment of epilepsy, hallucinations, obsessions and sexual overexcitation in people with mental disorders.

Blue crystals and minerals are good for febrile conditions, including those caused by infectious diseases.

Blue and cyan colors deservedly have a reputation for remarkable antiseptics, which have long been used as a disinfectant.

In folk medicine, stones such as lapis lazuli, turquoise, aquamarine have always been used to correct myopia and treat various eye diseases, including serious ones like corneal damage, glaucoma, and cataracts.

Blue and cyan stones help with liver diseases (including hepatitis), joints, and rheumatic diseases. They are recommended by stone therapists for neurological pain, diseases of the spine, including osteochondrosis.

Blue and cyan stones have a certain specialization. For example, lapis lazuli has been used for many centuries to treat eye diseases and some skin diseases. The powder from it was used in folk medicine of different countries to cleanse the body of toxins. He was considered one of the most effective antidotes.

It is also believed that sapphires, blue tourmalines, and topazes are very effective for normalizing the activity of the endocrine system of the body. Accordingly, their use is recommended for pathologies of the thyroid gland.

Amazonites, azurites, blue topazes, tourmalines, opals, and agates are useful for cramping and headaches, fluorites, chalcedony, spinel, labradorites help with thyroid diseases. The crushed powder from azurite in the Middle Ages was used to remove bile from the body. Aquamarine has always been considered extremely useful for toothaches, as well as for relieving the feeling of heaviness in the stomach.

To reduce blood pressure, aquamarines, lapis lazuli, turquoise, and sapphires are indicated. They cannot only narrow blood vessels but also slow down the heartbeat and ease shortness of breath.

Turquoise, amazonites, blue sapphires, blue opals, spinel, hawkeye, labradors, sodalites have a positive effect in the treatment of inflammatory processes of the ear, throat, and nose. In addition, they are useful for relieving rheumatic pains.

Dark blue stones, such as azurites, iolites, sapphires, have a diverse and extremely effective effect on various lung diseases: they treat inflammatory processes of the respiratory tract, cleanse them of mucus, and help relieve shortness of breath and relieve spasms.

Almost all blue stones have a beneficial effect on headaches, especially spasmodic ones. In folk medicine in some eastern countries, blue and cyan minerals are often used for insect bites, burns, and also for the treatment of wounds of various origins. For example, the antiseptic properties of fluorites and chalcedony allow them to be used to heal tumors and wounds, including purulent ones.

Blue color is often used to rid children of various infections, fears, tics, stuttering, itching, and sleep disorders.

In gynecology, blue stones can make menstruation not only less painful but also less profuse. Regular contemplation of transparent blue gem stones is recommended to relieve tension of the premenstrual syndrome.

Purple Stones

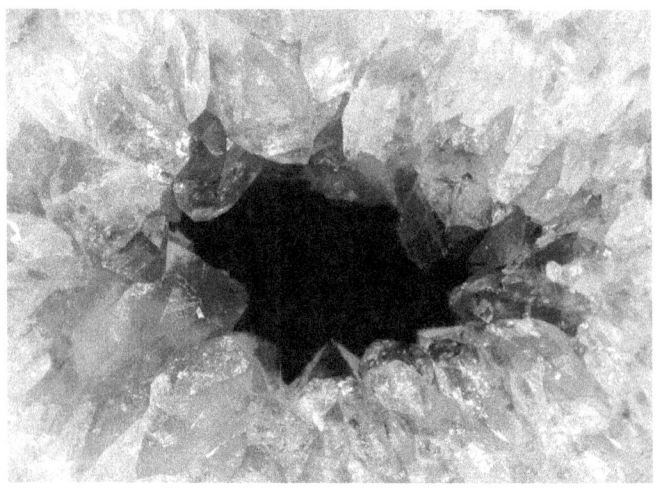

Amethysts, charoites, purple garnets (almandine), topazes, rubies, tourmalines, fluorites, spinel.

Violet and lilac colors have always been considered the colors of philosopher sages who know the truth of the meaning of being. Combining two strong colors - red and blue -purple is also a symbol of creation. It is interesting to note that modern research by scientists has shown that exposure to purple (naturally, in certain doses) increases the mental potential of a person.

The contemplation of beautiful stones and minerals, painted in different shades of purple and lilac tones, has a calming effect on the nervous system.

In nature, purple stones are quite rare. Perhaps that is why they have always been highly valued, including among the healers of different countries and peoples. People have long noticed that the color purple can have a powerful healing effect in the fight against a variety of ailments. It is especially often used for mental and nervous diseases, including those caused by various injuries (for example, concussion, severe psychological stress). Precious and semiprecious stones of violet and lilac shades also have a beneficial effect on improving working capacity, especially of people whose activities are associated with the creative process.

A remarkable effect is the use of purple minerals to improve the condition of people suffering from dementia and epilepsy. In folk medicine, the effectiveness of purple gems has long been observed in the treatment of neuralgia, joint pain, rheumatism, migraines, and the fight against insomnia. They are also recommended for colds and inflammatory processes.

Purple stones are used in the treatment of inflammatory processes of various origins. The most popular and most common among the stones of the violet spectrum in folk medicine is amethyst.

Beautiful delicate shades, most often lilac, have earned well-deserved fame for this amazing stone. It was recommended to be constantly worn by people who feel internal discomfort, anxiety, doubt. The powerful positive energy emanating from the amethyst is able to return the desired peace and inner harmony. It is also able to improve memory, strengthen mental activity.

White Stones

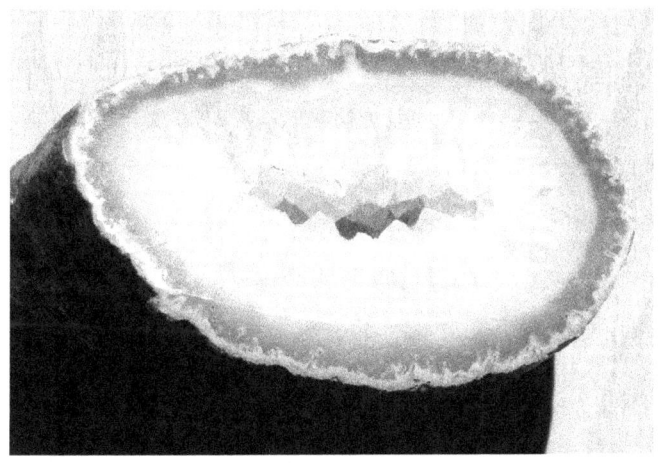

Diamond, adularia, colorless topazes, zircons and calcites (feldspars), rhinestone, white pearls, opals (cacholong), corals, cubic zirconias, jades, turquoise, milk quartz.

White color also embodies the spiritual strength and energy of healing. White stones for several millennia have been used by healers to improve the nervous system, musculoskeletal system (including tissue of the spinal cord and brain). Diamonds, cubic zirconias, rock crystal, milk quartz, and other white minerals remarkably cleanse the body of toxins and increase the vitality of the body.

Diamond in oriental medicine has been used for several millennia as a bleaching agent for removing age spots from the surface of the skin. In medieval treatises on medicine, the use of diamonds for the treatment of the effects of stroke and sclerosis, as well as for the prevention of kidney stones, is reported.

Transparent rhinestone is recommended to be worn on the right side of the abdomen for people suffering from pathologies of the gallbladder. In medieval Europe, doctors recommended it to increase the amount of milk for nursing mothers. Rhinestone helps eliminate bad breath and freshen breath.

In oriental medicine, pearls were widely used in hemoptysis, pathologies of the gastrointestinal tract, as well as an antispasmodic and tachycardia. Pearls of white color improve vision and help in the treatment of eye diseases.

Black Stones

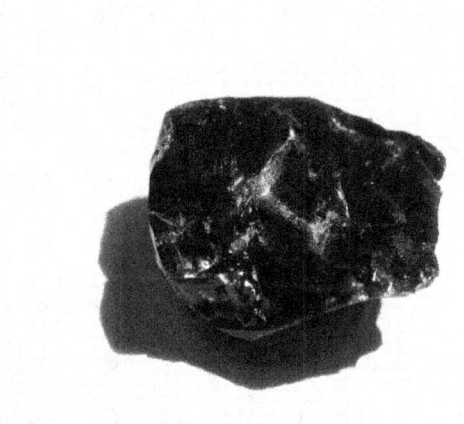

Hematite (blood), jet, morion, shungite, rauchtopaz, black agate, garnet, obsidian, jade, onyx, tourmaline, pearl, jasper.

Ferrous minerals contain powerful energy. In antiquity and the Middle Ages, they were considered symbols of wisdom, strength, courage. Using the energy of black stones for unseemly purposes was expensive for their owners. At the same time, they significantly facilitated the achievement of creative, noble goals, including such as the healing of people suffering from various bodily and spiritual ailments.

Black color remarkably contributes to the restoration of forces and harmonization of energy, especially among people whose professional activity is associated with high energy consumption, for example, public figures of different levels.

Some of them, such as jet, are effective for eye diseases. Others (hematites, obsidians) are used as a hemostatic agent. The jet was used in the early Middle Ages to treat gout.

Since the jet is a petrified wood, it was also used in the form of fumigation for people suffering from nervous diseases and epilepsy. Burnt and washed black coral has long been used by doctors as a means of strengthening the heart muscle and helping to interrupt its work.

Hematite, which after polishing acquires the color of dark clotted blood, was considered an effective hemostatic. It was also often used to treat diseases of the genitourinary system, especially in men.

Black stones in modern stone therapy have found application in the treatment of inflammation, tumors, diseases of the musculoskeletal system. Some of them (for example, rauchtopases) are used for bronchial asthma. Black stones are useful for eliminating skin diseases, healing wounds of various origins.

How to Work with Stones and Crystals in Reiki

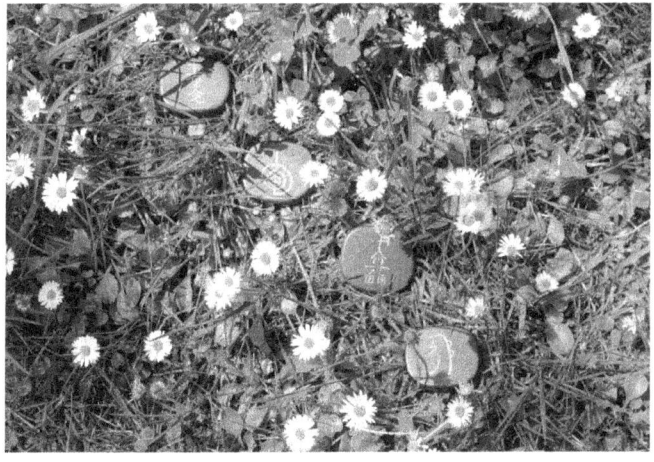

Before charging, the crystals are cleaned. This is necessary in order to free them from extraneous information. Stones perceive vibration and electromagnetic vibrations from the external environment, including from people, and thus can be polluted. If the treatment consists of wearing the crystal on the body, then it must be cleaned at least once a week. If the stone lies in the room and it is not always carried with you, then it is subjected to cleaning much less frequently.

The purification of crystals is carried out in various ways. They are placed for a day in salt water, for the same period they are covered with sea salt, and purified under running water. This method is also used for purification - each side of the crystal is blown with air and at the same time, it is imagined how the crystal becomes clean and transparent.

Crystals are also charged in various ways. For example, a crystal is left for several hours surrounded by other crystals or placed under a pyramid. This contributes to the concentration of energy within the crystal. Also, for charging, the crystals are immersed in colored solutions, they are exposed to light rays of different colors. You can charge the crystal, leaving it for a long time in an area with an amplified electromagnetic field. Crystals charge with the help of Reiki. The crystal is clamped between the palms and at the same time focus on the purpose for which it is intended.

The crystal can be charged mentally without touching it with your hands, sending healing units to it and then transferring it to the patient. You can hold the crystal in your hands and mentally send its energy to the patient while imagining how he takes it. The crystals perceive electromagnetic vibrations from the mentor and transmit them to their owners.

Crystals are natural resonators. They amplify the flow of energy from a Reiki master several times. That is why the effect of Reiki in combination with crystallotherapy is more effective. The crystal focuses the energy sent to it and directs it to the application area. Most often they are applied to the body in the area of the chakras.

Reiki affects many life processes and is used for various diseases, helps to overcome psychological problems, such as fears, denial of part of your personality, which contributes to spiritual growth and gaining mental maturity. Psychological problems often cause sleep disturbance, insecurity, decreased and loss of appetite, nightmares. Stones and crystals in combination with Reiki help get rid of these problems.

Crystals contribute to the treatment of bone fractures, wound healing, and pain management. They are used in the treatment of chronic diseases of internal organs, to restore the body after stress.

Stones and crystals help to improve well-being in various conditions associated not only with diseases. Stones of blue color help with heat, with fatigue and the desire to cheer up - yellow, if necessary, calm down - blue and lilac. Red stones will help get rid of a runny nose.

Under the influence of strong emotions and stress in the blood, the level of hormones rises sharply, which leads to metabolic disorders and provokes the accumulation of its by-products in the body and increases blood pressure. As a result, a prerequisite is created for the development of many diseases. Reiki in combination with crystals restores the energy system in the body and health.

After stress, it is recommended to conduct short Reiki sessions with crystals for several days. They are more effective than a long single exposure. During the session, the patient is recommended to sit or lie down. In these positions, you can relax and tune in to energy interaction with the healer and crystals.

On the chakra in the region of the heart, pink quartz is applied, which successfully relieves stress. Around it are four more crystals of pure quartz so that their vertices are directed diagonally relative to the midline of the body. Thus, they unlock the energy field in the region of the heart and prevent the accumulation of clots of negative energy in the subtle bodies.

A tiger eye is placed on the navel area where the sacral chakra is located. Around it, like pure quartz, rock crystal is placed. In the inguinal region and at the feet, grounding stones are laid out. These include the tiger eye, jasper, hematite, smoky quartz, carnelian, and magnetite. After the expressed stress is eliminated, the balance of the chakras is checked and the energy field is completely purified with the help of a crystal pendulum and massage rods. Of the crystals, jade, aventurine, amethyst, smoky quartz are suitable for this. Before this, the patient is recommended to drink water, which helps to cleanse the body.

Grounding enhances the perception of reality, it helps in focusing, improves memory, brings the body into a state of energy balance. Passive grounding is carried out in a sitting position. The crystals are placed on the front surface of the body in the sternum, in the inguinal region between the legs or between the feet and one is taken in each hand.

Your Energy Body – Energy Management

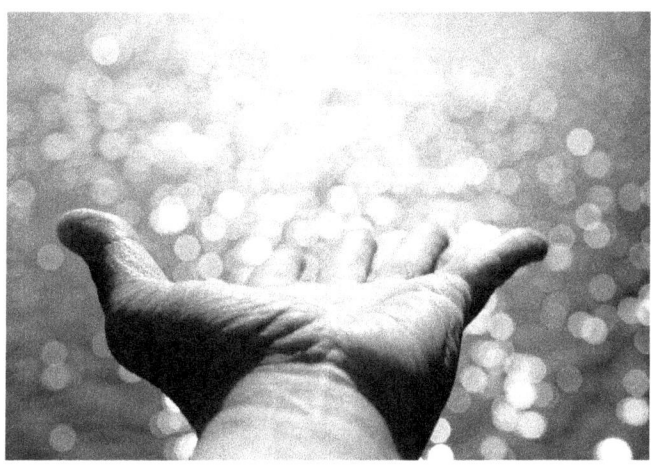

To quickly ground and strengthen the aura, smoky quartz is used. It is applied in the larynx. The second same crystal is placed in the lower back at the base of the spine so that it has a sharp end pointing toward the ground. For 10 minutes you need to be at rest and meditate, you can imagine yourself under the thin streams of a waterfall that wash the body from top to bottom. At this time, there is a release from negative emotions and pain.

Next, to harmonize the movement of energy through the channels, tap on the chest below the clavicles. After this, you can perform several breathing exercises, do yoga. After the classes, the feeling of heaviness disappears, calm and confidence appear.

Crystals and stones combined with Reiki help eliminate pain. Stones and crystals after charging are applied to a sore spot, then they are turned, not tearing off the surface of the body, in the counterclockwise direction. Thus, all negative energy leaves the body and is absorbed into the used object. After being removed from the body, the stone or crystal is shaken in the air, neutralizing the negative charge in it.

You can eliminate the pain in another way. A stone or crystal is taken in the left hand and tuned to the flow of energy emanating from it. It can be both positive and negative, it all depends on the direction of the used object. Then put the right palm to the sore spot and hold it there for 30 minutes.

10 REIKI - BIBLIOGRAPHY

To begin, I particularly recommend:

- ❖ Reiki Manuals I, II and III. Nita Mocanu. 2012 -2014.

  I thank N. Mocanu for all the information found in her Reiki handbooks and from which I have inspired myself to complete the Reiki pages.

- ❖ The Original Reiki Manual of Dr. Mikao Usui. Dr. Mikao Usui and Frank Arjava Petter. 2000.

  Very practical book in which Dr. Usui gives a

detailed description of the positions of the hands for the treatment of certain parts of the body and certain health problems.

- ❖ Reiki fire. Frank Arjava Petter. 1999.

- ❖ The Quintessence of Reiki. Walter Lubeck, Frank Arjava Petter, William Lee Rand. 2002.

In addition:

- ❖ The Complete Guide to Reiki. Tanmaya Honervogt. 2012.

- ❖ Reiki. The legacy of Dr. Usui. Frank Arjava Petter. 2000. Rediscovered documents on the origin and development of the Reiki system, as well as new aspects of Reiki Energy.

For those who want to deepen:

- ❖ Reiki - The most beautiful techniques. Walter Lubeck, Frank Arjava Petter. 2013.

- ❖ Japanese Reiki. Hand treatment with ease.

Mochizuki Toshitaka, Kaneko Miyuki. 2009

❖ Reiki manual. Frank Arjava Petter, Tadao Yamagushi, Churijo Hayashi. 2014.

Other books:

❖ The beneficial power of the hands. Barbara Ann Brennan. 1987.

  A very classic on energy techniques by the hands. A bit arduous…

❖ The quantum body. The fabulous healing powers of your mind. Dr. Deepak Chopra. 1990.

❖ The subtle body. The great encyclopedia of energy anatomy. Cyndi Dale. 2013.

❖ The harmony of energies Michel Odoul. 2002.

Tell me where you're hurting: I'll tell you why. Michel Odoul. 2002.

REIKI

CONCLUSION

A few years ago, my daughter came up to me and said: "Dad, I wonder what you are doing. I also want to try." Then she was twelve years old.

I opened to her some points on the meridians and activated the seventh, sixth and fourth chakras. After a couple of months, she admitted that she sometimes began to see the internal organs of people. When I asked her to look at my internal organs, she said that she could not, because they are well-protected ki, and she sees only a swirling light fog. Then I tested it, concentrating my ki in different energy fields or transferring it to different parts of my body. She correctly identified the places of energy accumulation. Now the daughter can even see how electric current flows along the "wires".

My daughter's spiritual vision is very helpful in diagnosing diseases. I do not own such a gift. She can say exactly what the internal organs are affected because the diseased organ is surrounded by dark ki. When I passed Reiki to my patients, Alexandra saw a bright golden stream flowing from somewhere above, from my hands, from my head and dispersing dark spots around the diseased organs. In general, spiritual development in children is much faster than in adults. By the way, almost all women at the third level of our school become "seeing".

I have two possible explanations for this phenomenon. Firstly, according to modern science, the spectrum of electromagnetic radiation has a wavelength of 0.000000047 microns to 30 km. But the range visible by the eyes is very small - from 0.4 to 0.8 microns (0.0004-0.0008 mm)! By practicing Reiki, you can expand this limited range and acquire the ability to see things that an ordinary person cannot see.

Secondly, our eyes, like other organs, are just tools of the mind. In fact, we see with the mind, not with the eyes. My daughter, as a result of Reiki studies, began to perceive with an inner gaze what is inaccessible to the ordinary eye. She told me about cases when she could not clearly see the subject. Then she concentrated the mind, and a clear mental picture arose.

You can achieve this, alongside with healing. Reiki is available for all, and for you. You just have to set your sights, and your heart, on achieving (attainments and attunements) at its highest levels!

www.ingramcontent.com/pod-product-compliance
Lightning Source LLC
Chambersburg PA
CBHW060833220526
45466CB00003B/1086